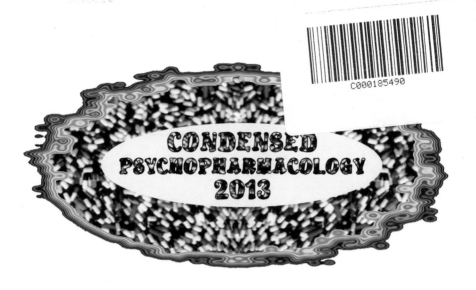

CONDENSED PSYCHOPHARMACOLOGY 2013

A Pocket Reference for Psychiatry and Psychotropic Medications

By:
Leonard Rappa, PharmD, BCPP
Professor, Florida A&M University
College of Pharmacy and Pharmaceutical Sciences
Board Certified Psychiatric Pharmacist
Licensed Consultant Pharmacist
Fort Lauderdale, Florida

Contributing Author:
James Viola, PharmD, BCPP
Clinical Pharmacist, Mental Health-Veterans Administration
Adjunct Clinical Assistant Professor of Pharmacy
University of Florida
Board Certified Psychiatric Pharmacist

Published by RXPSYCH LLC, Ft. Lauderdale, FL
© December 2012

TABLE OF CONTENTS

Background Information for Psychiatry 1

Commonly Used Psychiatric Terms and Abbreviations 2

General Psychotropic Medication Information 3

Black Box Warnings 5

Time Frame for Medications to Show Efficacy 6

Key Drug Levels 7

Diseases of Significance 7

Delirium Acronym 7

Clinically Significant Drug Interactions 7

Evidence-Based Medicine 8

Drugs That Mimic or Cause Cognitive Impairment 8

Anticholinergic Activity of Frequently Used Medications 8

Active Metabolites and Enantiomers 8

Metabolites Which Are Marketed as Other Drugs 8

Psychiatric Medications: Important Side Effects and Monitoring Parameters 9

Triggers of Depression and Triggers of Anxiety 10

Non-Addictive Treatments of Pain and Insomnia 11

Common DSM-IV TR Personality Disorders in Psychiatric Patients 12

Attention Deficit Hyperactivity Disorder 13

Amphetamine Comparison Chart 14

Bipolar Medications (Anti-Manics / Mood Stabilizers) 15

Major Depression and Antidepressants 17

Antidepressants' Mechanism of Action Explained 20

Common Antidepressant Side Effects 21

Serotonin Syndrome 22

Anxiolytics and PTSD 23

Comparison of Common Benzodiazepines 24

Antipsychotics (Neuroleptics / Major Tranquilizers) 25

Treatment of EPS 25

Risk of Metabolic Syndrome, QTc Prolongation, Prolactin Elevations, and Dose-related EPS with Atypical Antipsychotics 29

Antipsychotic Charts and Pearls 29

Long Acting Injectable Chart 30

Substance-Related Disorders 31

Intoxication / Detoxification Information 32

Effects at Specific Blood Alcohol Concentrations 33

Urine Detection of Drugs 34

Opioid Comparison Chart (Equianalgesic Dosing) 35

Special Populations and Issues in Psychiatry 36

Possible Pharmacotherapeutic Interventions 38

References 39

Index 46

BACKGROUND INFORMATION FOR PSYCHIATRY

A. **DSM-IV-TR**
The Diagnostic and Statistical Manual of Mental Disorders (DSM-IV TR) in its 4th edition, text revised.[1]
It is published by the American Psychiatric Association and provides diagnostic criteria for mental disorders. Time frames for diagnoses and required symptoms are included.

B. **MULTI-AXIAL DIAGNOSIS**
1. Axis I: Main psychiatric diagnosis
2. Axis II: Personality Disorders or Mental Retardation
3. Axis III: Co-morbid medical disorders (supposedly related to psychiatric diagnosis)
4. Axis IV: Psychosocial stressors (listed)
   a. i.e. Divorce, school issues, job-related stress
5. Axis V: Global Assessment of Functioning (GAF)
   a. Scale of function from 0 to 100 (0=lowest / 100=highest)
   b. See DSM-IV TR book for more information

C. **BAKER ACT (Florida Mental Health Act of 1971) - SPECIFIC TO FLORIDA!**
1. Definition: A law that protects the patient's rights while in a psychiatric hospital
   A. Florida Statutes – Chapter 394 (summary can be found at:
   http://www.floridasupremecourt.org/pub_info/documents/BakerSummary.pdf)
2. Many states have very analogous laws about mental health patients, so many of these terms and definitions may be similar in other states.
3. Terminology:
   A. Consent to treatment – Patient agrees to be in the hospital
      1. The capacity of a patient to understand and agree is up to psychiatrist
      2. If psychiatrist deems patient not able to give expressed and informed consent, a Proxy or Guardian Advocate must be found
   B. Consent for medication
      1. Patient is informed of purposes of prescribed medication, common side effects, risks, and alternatives to medication
      2. Even if patients is admitted involuntarily, he/she can consent or not consent to medications
      3. A patient is never force-medicated if no consent is given, unless in the event of an emergency or a guardian or judge gives permission
   C. Typical Baker Act – Involuntary hospitalization for up to 72 hours by law enforcement or the judicial system (Time can be extended by a court hearing)
   D. Voluntary Admission
      1. Patient consents to treatment or admitting self to hospital setting
   E. Application for Discharge (FL Statute Section 394.4625(2))
      1. If a patient is hospitalized and voluntarily consents to treatment, then he/she may revoke consent at any time. The attending psychiatrist has up to 24 hours to discharge the patient AMA (Against Medical Advice) or making the patient involuntary (becomes Baker-Acted and goes to court)
   F. Marchman Act: An involuntary admission due to substance abuse Impairment
      1. See Chapter 397 of the Florida Statutes
   G. Emergency Treatment Orders (ETOs)
      1. If a patient is deemed by their psychiatrist to be unable to consent to treatment or medications, and a guardian or proxy cannot be obtained in a timely manner, the physician treats the patient based on these ETOs (only valid for 24 hours each)
   H. Guardian Advocate or Proxy
      1. Assigned when a patient is deemed unable to consent to treatment to protect the patient's rights and consent for medications
   I. Court-ordered detainment
      1. After the 72hr period of the Baker Act is up, a psychiatrist must either let the patient go or petition the court for more time to treat the patient (involuntarily) – Petition must be filed before the BA expires (w/in 72hrs)
      2. The court can decide to let the patient go, or decide to retain them for an indeterminate amount of time for treatment
      3. The patient can still refuse medication if capable of consenting unless court-ordered to be force-medicated. A Guardian Advocate can consent for medications at this point, even against the patient's will.

D. **MEDICATION ALGORITHMS**
1. Texas Medication Algorithm Project (official site with algorithms etc), Texas Department of State Health Services - Best Practices Clearinghouse for Mental Health Systems
   http://www.dshs.state.tx.us/mhsa/clearinghouse/
2. The National Guideline Clearinghouse™ - U.S. Department of Health & Human Services - Agency for Healthcare Research and Quality
   http://www.guideline.gov (searchable for all treatments)

COMMONLY USED PSYCHIATRIC TERMS AND ABBREVIATIONS
(unless otherwise defined herein)

- 5HT – Serotonin
- ADD / ADHD – Attention Deficit Disorder / Hyperactivity Disorder
- AMA – Against Medical Advice
- BA – Baker Act
- BBW – Black Box Warning
- BPAD - Bipolar Affective Disorder
- BPD - Borderline Personality Disorder (Some clinicians use as Bipolar D/O so caution)
- BUN – Blood Urea Nitrogen
- BZD – Benzodiazepine
- C/O – Complains of
- CBC – Complete Blood Count
- CBZ – Carbamazepine
- CNS – Central Nervous System
- CR – Controlled Release
- CV – Cardiovascular
- CXR – Chest X-Ray
- D/O – Disorder
- D/T – Due to
- DA or D – Dopamine
- DCF – Department of Children and Families
- Def. – Deferred
- Diff – Differential
- DJJ – Department of Juvenile Justice
- DT – Delirium Tremens
- EKG – Electro Cardiogram
- EP – Elopement Precautions
- EPS – Extrapyramidal Side Effects
- ETO – Emergency Treatment Order
- FAS – Fetal Alcohol Syndrome
- FDA – Food and Drug Administration
- GABA – Gamma Aminobutyric Acid
- GAD – Generalized Anxiety Disorder
- GI – Gastrointestinal
- H&P – History and Physical
- H/I – Homicidal Ideation
- H_1 – Histamine 1 receptor
- HIV – Human Immunodeficiency Virus
- HTN – Hypertension
- IM – Intramuscular
- MA – Marchman Act
- MAO / MAOI – Monoamine Oxidase / Inhibitor

- MDD – Major Depressive Disorder
- MOA – Mechanism of Action
- MR – Mental Retardation
- MSE - Mental Status Exam
- MMSE - Mini Mental Status Exam
- N/V – Nausea and Vomiting
- NE – Norepinephrine
- NOS – None Otherwise Specified
- OCD – Obsessive Compulsive Disorder
- OCPD-Obsessive Compulsive Personality Disorder
- OOB – Up and out of bed
- OROS – Osmotically Controlled Release Oral Delivery System
- P450 – Cytochrome P450 enzyme system
- PD - Panic Disorder or Personality Disorder
- PMS / PMDD – Premenstrual Syndrome / Dysphoric Disorder
- prn – As needed
- PSA – Polysubstance Abuse
- QD / BID / TID / QID / HS – Daily / 2X a day / 3X a day / 4X a day / Bedtime
- RR – Regular Release
- Ψ - Psi – Unapproved abbreviation for PSYCH
- S/I – Suicidal Ideation
- SAD – Seasonal Affective Disorder (depends on location)
- SAD – Schizoaffective Disorder (Schizophrenia + Bipolar/mood component)
- SCAD – Schizoaffective Disorder
- SCPT – Schizophrenia Paranoid Type
- SCUD – Schizophrenia Undifferentiated
- SIADH – Syndrome of Inappropriate Antidiuretic Hormone
- SP – Suicide Precautions
- SSRI – Selective Serotonin Reuptake Inhibitor
- SNRI-Serotonin Norepinephrine Reuptake Inhibitor
- SZ – Seizure Precautions
- TB – Tuberculosis
- TCA – Tricyclic Antidepressant
- Tx. – Treatment
- UNSPEC – Unspecified
- VPA – Valproic Acid
- WBC – White Blood Cells
- XR or ER – Extended Release

GENERAL PSYCHOTROPIC MEDICATION INFORMATION

ANTIDEPRESSANTS:

Generic Name	Brand Name	Usual Adult Daily Dose	Other Indications/Uses
Amitriptyline[α]	Elavil®* Metabolized to	25-300 mg	Nocturnal Enuresis
Imipramine[α]	Tofranil®**	25-300 mg	Anxiety
Doxepin[α]	Sinequan®, Adapin®	25-300 mg	OCD
Trimipramine[α]	Surmontil®	25-300 mg	Panic Disorder
Clomipramine[α]	Anafranil®	25-250 mg	Neuropathic pain

(TCA / Tertiary amines / 5HT > NE)

Nortriptyline[α]	Pamelor®*	25-200 mg	Insomnia
Desipramine[α]	Norpramin®**	25-300 mg	
Protriptyline[α]	Vivactil®	15-60 mg	Headaches

(TCA / Secondary amines / NE > 5HT)

Amoxapine[α]	Asendin®	50-600 mg	
Maprotiline[α]	Ludiomil®	50-225 mg	
Phenelzine[α]	Nardil®	15-90 mg	Anxiety
Tranylcypromine[α]	Parnate®	10-60 mg	Psychotic depression
Selegiline[α]	Emsam®	6-12 mg (patch)	Depression
Isocarboxazid[α]	Marplan®	20-60 mg	Depression
Fluoxetine[α]	Prozac®/Sarafem®	20-80mg	OCD/Bulimia/PMDD
Sertraline[α]	Zoloft®	50-200mg	Panic Disorder / Anxiety
Paroxetine[α]	Paxil®/CR®/Pexeva®	20-50mg	Premature Ejaculation
Fluvoxamine[α]	Luvox®/CR®	50-300mg	Headaches/PMDD/OCD
Citalopram[α,β]	Celexa®	20-40mg	PTSD
Escitalopram[α]	Lexapro®	10-20mg	Anxiety Disorders
Vilazodone[α]	Viibryd™	10-40mg (with food)	
Trazodone[α]	Desyrel®/Oleptro™	50-450mg	Insomnia
Nefazodone[α,χ]	Serzone®	100-600mg	Anxious depression
Bupropion[α]/Budeprion®	Wellbutrin®/Aplenzin®/Forfivo™XL	75-450mg (÷TID)	ADHD /Smoking (Zyban®)
Venlafaxine[α]	Effexor/XR®***	37.5-375mg	Neuropathic pain
Duloxetine[α]	Cymbalta®	20-120mg/d	Diabetic neuropathy, GAD, Fibromyalgia
Desvenlafaxine[α]	Pristiq™***	50-100mg/d	
Mirtazapine[α]	Remeron®/Sol-tab®	15-45mg (at HS)	Insomnia, ↑ appetite
Milnacipran[α]	Savella®	12.5-200mg/d(÷BID)	Fibromyalgia

* and ** and *** antidepressants are metabolized to the other (following the arrows)
α,β,χ - *See Black Box Warnings on Page 5*

MOOD STABILIZERS / ANTICONVULSANTS:

Generic Name	Brand Name	Usual Daily Dose)	Other Indications/Uses
Lithium[δ]	Eskalith®, Lithobid®	300-2700	Cluster headache, Bipolar
Carbamazepine[ε,φ]	Tegretol®/XR, Epitol®, Equetro™, Carbatrol®	200-1200	Aggression, Epilepsy, Bipolar Disorder, Peripheral Neuropathy
Valproic Acid[γ,η,ι]	Depakote®/ER/Stavzor® Depakene® / Depacon®	500-3000	Epilepsy, Migraine Headaches, Hiccups
Lamotrigine	Lamictal®	50-500	Epilepsy, Bipolar maintenance
Olanzapine + fluoxetine	Symbyax®[α,κ]	3/25 to 12/50	Bipolar depression
Phenobarbital	Luminal®	30-240	Epilepsy, Drug withdrawal
Primidone	Mysoline®/Sertan®	100-2000	Epilepsy
Ethosuximide	Zarontin®	500-1500	Epilepsy
Felbamate	Felbatol®	1200-3600	Epilepsy
Gabapentin	Neurontin®/Gralise®	900-1800	Epilepsy, ALS, neuralgias
Phenytoin[μ]	Dilantin®	50-400	Epilepsy
Topiramate	Topamax®	50-1600÷bid (avg=200mg bid)	Epilepsy, Migraine
Oxcarbazepine	Trileptal®/Oxtellar XR®	300-2400÷bid (4-16yrs old: 8-10mg/kg/d ÷bid/tid up to 1800mg/d)	
Tiagabine	Gabitril®	4-56 ÷bid/qid (children: 2-32mg/d ÷bid/qid) Epilepsy	
Zonisamide	Zonegran®	100-600 ÷bid	
Levetiracetam	Keppra®/XR®	1000-3000 ÷bid	
Clobazam	Onfi®	5-40mg (note: C-IV BZD–for Lennox Gastaut Syndrome – ages 2 & up)	

δ,ε,φ,γ,η,ι,φ,α,κ,λ,μ - *See Black Box Warnings on Page 5*

PSYCHOSTIMULANTS / ADHD MEDICATIONS (FOR FULL LIST SEE PAGE 14):

Generic Name	Brand Name	Usual Daily Dose	Other Uses
Dextroamphetamine[ν]	Dexedrine®	5-60mg	Wt loss, Narcolepsy
Methylphenidate[ν]	Ritalin® / Daytrana™	5-60mg	Weight loss
	Concerta® / Metadate® / Methylin®/ Focalin®		Narcolepsy
Lisdexamfetamine[ν]	Vyvanse™	20-70mg/d	
4 amphetamine salts:	Adderall®/ XR[ν]	2.5-40mg	Weight loss
(Dextroamphetamine saccharate, Amphetamine aspartate, Dextroamphetamine sulfate, Amphetamine sulfate)			
Modafinil[α]	Provigil®/Sparlon®	85-225mg /d	Narcolepsy
Atomoxetine[α]	Strattera™	0.5mg/kg/day up to 1.4mg/kg/day or 100mg/day	
Clonidine	Catapres®/Kapvay™	0.05mg up to 25mcg/kg/day	HTN/Tics/Tourette's
Guanfacine	Tenex® / Intuniv™	1-4mg/d	HTN/Tics/Tourette's

α,ν - *See Black Box Warnings on Page 5*

TYPICAL ANTIPSYCHOTICS:

Generic Name	Brand Name	Usual Daily Dose	Other Indications/Uses
Chlorpromazine[κ]	Thorazine®	25-1600mg	Hiccups/Bipolar/Dementia/Anxiety/N&V/Agitation
Thioridazine[κ,β]	Mellaril® Metab. to	10-800mg	Anxiety/Agitation
Mesoridazine[κ,β]	Serentil®	10-300mg	Nausea / vomiting/Agitation
Molindone[κ]	Moban®	10-100mg	
Loxapine[κ]	Loxitane®/Adasuve®	10-100mg	Agitation
Perphenazine[κ]	Trilafon®	2-64mg	N/V/Acute psychosis/psychotic depression /hiccups/Agitation
Trifluoperazine[κ]	Stelazine®	1-30mg	Anxiety
Thiothixene[κ]	Navane®	2-30mg	Acute psychosis/Agitation/Psychotic depression
Fluphenazine[κ]	Prolixin®	1-40mg	Acute psychosis/Psychotic depression/Agitation
Haloperidol[κ]	Haldol®	0.5-40mg	Acute psychosis/ADHD/Tourette's/ Agitation/ Autism/Delirium/Migraine/N/V /Hiccups

κ,β - See Black Box Warnings on Page 5

OLDER COMBINATION PRODUCTS:

Generic Name	Brand Name	Usual Daily Dose	Other Indications/Uses
Perphenazine + amitriptyline[α,κ]	Triavil®	2/10, 4/10, 2/25, 4/25, 4/50 up to QID	anxiety, psychotic
Perphenazine + amitriptyline[α,κ]	Etrafon®, Etrafon-A®	2/10, 2/25, 4/10 up to QID	depression, schizo.
Chlordiazepoxide+amitriptyline[α,κ]	Limbitrol®, Limbitrol DS®	5/12.5, 10/25 up to QID	anxiety, depression

α,κ - See Black Box Warnings on Page 5

ATYPICAL ANTIPSYCHOTICS:

Generic Name	Brand Name	Usual Daily Dose	Other Indications/Uses
Clozapine[κ,ο,π,θ,ρ]	Clozaril®, Fazaclo®	25-900mg	Tx. Resistant schizo./SCAD/BPAD /agitation/tremor
Risperidone*♦ metabolized to	Risperdal®/M-Tabs®κ Risperdal® Consta®	1-16mg	Autism/ADHD/psychotic depression /Tourette's Syndrome/ Agitation/ Acute psychosis
Paliperidone*♦	Invega®κ / Sustenna®	6-12mg	SCAD
Ziprasidone*	Geodon®κ (÷ bid)	20-160mg (w/food)	Agitation/Acute psychosis/Tourette's
Quetiapine*♦	Seroquel®/XR®α,κ	25-800mg	Bipolar Depression/Adjunct for MDD/ Agitation/Acute Psychosis/OCD
Olanzapine*♦	Zyprexa®/Zydis®κ,σ/Relprevv™	2.5-20mg	Agitation/Acute psychosis
Olanzapine/Fluoxetine (OFC®α,κ or Symbyax®)		3/25-12/50mg	Treatment Resistant Depression
Aripiprazole*♦+	Abilify®α,κ	10-30mg	Adjunct for MDD/Agitation/Autism/ Acute psychosis
Iloperidone	Fanapt®κ	12-24mg (divided bid)	
Asenapine*	Saphris®κ SL tabs	10-20mg (divided bid)	
Lurasidone	Latuda®κ	40-160mg/d (with FOOD)	

♦Approved in children &/or adolescents /*Approved for Bipolar Disorder/*Approved as add-on therapy in depression

α,κ,ο,π,θ,ρ,σ - See Black Box Warnings on Page 5

NON-BENZODIAZEPINE SEDATIVE AGENTS:

Generic name	Brand name	FDA-Approved for Sleep	Usual dosage range (mg/d)[a]	Other Uses
Zolpidem	Ambien®/CR®/Intermezzo	Yes	2.5-10	
Zaleplon	Sonata®	Yes	5-20	
Eszopiclone	Lunesta™	Yes	1-3	
Ramelteon	Rozerem®	Yes	8	
Diphenhydramine	Benadryl®	Yes	25-200	Allergy
Doxylamine	Nyquil®	Yes	25-50	
Doxepin[α]	Silenor®	Yes	3-6	
Trazodone[κ]	Desyrel®	No	25-150	Depression
Hydroxyzine pamoate	Vistaril®	No	50-400	Agitation
Hydroxyzine HCL	Atarax®	No	10-30	Allergy/itch
Meprobamate	Equanil®, Miltown®	No	400-1600	Anticonvulsant

NON-BENZODIAZEPINE ANTI-ANXIETY AGENTS:

Generic name	Brand name	Approved for Anxiety	Usual dosage range (mg/d)[a]	Other Uses
Hydroxyzine pamoate	Vistaril®	Yes	50-400	Agitation
Hydroxyzine HCL	Atarax®	No		Allergy/itching
Meprobamate	Equanil®/Miltown®	Yes	400-1600	Anticonvulsant
Propranolol[τ]	Inderal®	No	80-160	Impulsivity/Aggression
Buspirone	Buspar®/ Dividose®	Yes	15-60	

α,τ - See Black Box Warnings on Page 5

BENZODIAZEPINES:

Generic name	Brand name	FDA Approved indications	Approved dosage range (mg/d)[a]	Approved equivalent dose (mg)
Alprazolam	Xanax®/XR®	Anxiety / Panic disorder	0.75-10	0.5
	Niravam®	Anxiety-depression		
Chlordiazepoxide	Librium®	Anxiety / Alcohol withdrawal	25-200	25
Clonazepam	Klonopin®	Panic disorder / Seizures	0.125-20	0.25
Clorazepate	Tranxene®	Anxiety / Seizure disorders	7.5-90	10
Diazepam	Valium®	Anxiety / Alcohol withdrawal	2-40	5
Estazolam	ProSom®	Sedative-Hypnotic	1-2	1
Halazepam	Paxipam®	Anxiety	20-160	20
Lorazepam	Ativan®	Anxiety / Pre-op sedation	0.5-10	1
Oxazepam	Serax®	Anxiety / Anxiety-depression Alcohol withdrawal	30-120	15
Prazepam	Centrax®	Anxiety	20-60	10
Temazepam	Restoril®	Sedative-Hypnotic	15-30	10
Triazolam	Halcion®	Sedative-Hypnotic	0.125-0.25	0.25

[a] Elderly patients are usually treated with approximately one-half of the dose listed

ALZHEIMER'S MEDICATIONS:

Generic name	Brand name	Dosage forms available	Dosage range (mg/d)
Donepezil	Aricept®	Tablet, orally disintegrating tablet	5-23mg QAM
Rivastigmine	Exelon®	Capsule, solution (2mg/ml), patch	1.5-6mg po BID or 4.6-9.5mg/24h patch
Galantamine	Razadyne®/ER®	Tablet, solution (4mg/ml), ER capsule	8-32mg (÷bid for IR forms)
Memantine	Namenda®	Tablet, solution (2mg/ml)	5-20mg ÷ bid when can

BLACK BOX WARNINGS

α - Suicidality and Antidepressant Drugs - Antidepressants increased the risk compared to placebo of suicidal thinking and behavior (suicidality) in children, adolescents, and young adults in short-term studies of Major Depressive Disorder (MDD) and other psychiatric disorders. Anyone considering the use of an antidepressant in a child, adolescent, or young adult must balance this risk with the clinical need. Short-term studies did not show an increase in the risk of suicidality with antidepressants compared to placebo in adults beyond age 24; there was a reduction in risk with antidepressants compared to placebo in adults aged 65 and older. Depression and certain other psychiatric disorders are themselves associated with increases in the risk of suicide.

β - Non-Black Box Warning: Proarrhythmic Effects - QT-Prolongation and *Torsades de Pointes*

χ - Cases of life-threatening hepatic failure have been reported

δ - Lithium toxicity is closely related to its serum levels and can occur at dose close to therapeutic levels

ε - Serious dermatologic reactions and HLA-B*1502 Allele - including toxic epidermal necrolysis and Stevens-Johnson syndrome; the risk is 10x greater in Asian countries; the allele is almost exclusively in Asian patients

φ - Aplastic Anemia/Agranulocytosis - the risk of developing these conditions are 5-8x higher than the general population

γ - Hepatoxicity - hepatic failure has been reported especially during the first six month of therapy. Hepatic failure is at a considerably increase risk in children

η - Teratogenicity - valproate can produce teratogenic effect such neural tube defects

ι - Pancreatitis - cases of life threatening pancreatitis has been reported in both children and adult

ο - Serious Rashes - Serious rashes including Stevens-Johnson syndrome may occur requiring hospitalization and discontinuation of treatment

κ - Dementia-Related Psychosis - elderly patients with dementia-related psychosis treated with antipsychotic drugs are at an increased risk of death; not approved for the treatment of patients with dementia-related psychosis

λ - Aplastic Anemia - Felbatol should only be use in patient whose epilepsy is so severe that the risk of aplastic anemia is acceptable in light of the benefit; also a patient should be on therapy without proper hematologic

μ - Cardiovascular Risk with Rapid Infusion - infusion should not exceed 50 mg/min (adults) or 1-3 mg/kg/min whichever is slower (peds pts); incr. risk of severe hypotension and cardiac arrhythmias above recommended infusion rate

ν - High Abuse Potential, Dependency - high abuse potential; avoid prolonged tx, may lead to drug dependence; potential for non-therapeutic use or distribution to others; prescribe/dispense sparingly; serious cardiovascular adverse events and sudden death reported w/ misuse

ο - Agranulocytosis

π - Seizures

θ - Myocarditis

ρ - Other cardiovascular and respiratory effects (orthostatic hypotension, respiratory/cardiac arrest, collapse)

σ - Patients are at risk for severe sedation (including coma) and/or delirium after each injection and must be observed for at least 3 hours in a registered facility with ready access to emergency response services.

τ - Avoid Abrupt Cessation - severe angina exacerbation, MI, and ventricular arrhythmias in angina pts after abrupt D/C; taper gradually over 1-2 weeks and monitor when D/C

TIME FRAME FOR MEDICATIONS TO SHOW EFFICACY

ANTIDEPRESSANTS
- ❖ Generally 2-6 weeks for maximum antidepressant efficacy, but may be up to 12 weeks[2,3,4]
  - ➤ Early switching to another agent may not benefit patient more than waiting[5]
- ❖ No drug is proven to take full effect faster than another, with the exception of mirtazapine[6]
  - ➤ Exactly how much faster mirtazapine works is unknown, but it ↑ risks of weight gain
- ❖ Some symptoms may improve in first few days to 1 week, but signs and symptoms are still there

ANTIPSYCHOTICS[7,8,9]
Typical:
- ➤ 1-2 days: hyperactivity, combativeness, hostility
- ➤ 1-2 weeks: hallucinations, sleep, appetite, hygiene, delusions, social skills
- ➤ 1-2 months: judgment, insight

Atypical
- ➤ Effects on negative symptoms and cognition may take months

ANXIOLYTICS[10,11]
Benzodiazepines: Usual onset from 10 minutes up to 1-2 hours
- ➤ Onset depends upon absorptive, distributive, and lipophilic properties of individual drug
  - ◆ Rapid: Diazepam, Clorazepate, Alprazolam
  - ◆ Intermediate: Chlordiazepoxide, Lorazepam
  - ◆ Slow: Prazepam, Oxazepam, Temazepam, Clonazepam

Buspirone: 5HT1a partial agonist[12]
- ➤ Anxiolytic onset in 10-14 days
- ➤ Not a prn drug

MOOD STABILIZERS / ANTIMANIC AGENTS[13,14,15]
Lithium: 7 to 14 days for onset of efficacy / maximal efficacy in 1 month

Carbamazepine and Valproic Acid
- ➤ Onset in first "several days" to weeks
- ➤ Maximal efficacy when steady state blood levels reach higher spectrum of therapeutic range

For Acute Mania
- ➤ Antipsychotic drugs are more effective than mood stabilizers
  - ◆ In order of efficacy: Risperidone > Olanzapine > Haloperidol
  - ◆ From 68 randomized controlled trials of 16,073 patients[16]

Key Drug Levels[17,18,19,20,21,22,23]
-- Must wait 3-7 days after a dosage change or it may not be accurate
-- Draw level first thing in the AM before giving a dose

Lithium	→ 0.4 – 1.2 mEq/L
Valproic Acid	→ 50 – 125 mcg/ml
Carbamazepine	→ 4 – 12 mcg/ml
Phenytoin	→ 10 – 20 mcg/ml
Phenobarbital	→ 15 – 40 mcg/ml
Nortriptyline	→ 50 – 150 ng/ml
Desipramine	→ 125 – 300 ng/ml

DISEASES OF SIGNIFICANCE

Parkinson's Disease - high depression risk
- Approx. 40% comorbidity
- Parkinson's medications can ↑ risk of psychosis

Alzheimer's Disease - high depression risk
- Atypical antipsychotics ↑ risk of death by 1.7X
- Avoid benzodiazepines and anticholinergic drugs

Crohn's Disease - high comorbid anxiety

Infectious diseases (TB, Hepatitis C, HIV, Syphilis, Encephalitis) - high depression/psychosis risk

UTIs and Upper Respiratory Infections – may cause psychosis (especially in the elderly)

Dialysis – psychosis and mood lability
See www.renalpharmacyconsultants.com for dialysis help

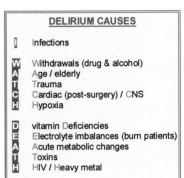

DELIRIUM CAUSES

0 Infections

W Withdrawals (drug & alcohol)
A Age / elderly
T Trauma
C Cardiac (post-surgery) / CNS
H Hypoxia

D vitamin Deficiencies
E Electrolyte imbalances (burn patients)
A Acute metabolic changes
T Toxins
H HIV / Heavy metal

CLINICALLY SIGNIFICANT DRUG INTERACTIONS

Linezolid (Zyvox®)[24] - This antibiotic is a monoamine oxidase inhibitor (MAOI)
- -Combined with an SSRI, TCA, or other MAOI can increase the risk of serotonin syndrome or hypertensive crisis

Ziprasidone (Geodon®)[25] **or Iloperidone (Fanapt®)**[26]
- Contraindicated if combined with other QT-prolonging drugs such as quinidine, thioridazine, moxifloxacin and many others (see www.qtdrugs.org for more information)
- Normal QTc should be < 420-440ms
   - o NOTE: QTc is not the same as QT
      - QTc is a corrected value that adjusts for factors such as heart rate
   - o A high QTc in males is >450ms and in females >470ms
- EKGs should be performed before therapy begins and after the end dose is reached
- A prolonged QT interval is a risk factor for ventricular tachyarrhythmia, *torsades de pointes*, and sudden death

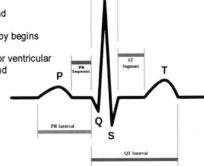

Image courtesy of http://en.wikipedia.org/wiki/File:SinusRhythmLabels.svg

EVIDENCE-BASED MEDICINE: Using the strongest medical evidence based on scientific studies to make appropriate pharmacotherapy decisions.

- Trileptal® (oxcarbazepine) OR Topamax® (topiramate) OR Neurontin® (gabapentin)
  - Not effective as monotherapy versus placebo in children or adults with Bipolar Disorder[27,28]
- Antipsychotic polypharmacy does not increase therapy's initial effectiveness
  - Antipsychotic polypharmacy may increase the risk for diabetes and the metabolic syndrome[29,30,31,32,33]

DRUGS THAT MIMIC OR CAUSE COGNITIVE IMPAIRMENT

• Anticholinergics	• Skeletal Muscle Relaxants	• Digoxin
• Antihistamines	• Anticonvulsants	• Disopyramide
• Sedative/hypnotics	• Antipsychotics	• Lithium
• Narcotics	• Antiemetics	• Cimetidine
• Corticosteroids	• Antidepressants	• Indomethacin
• Antiparkinsonian agents	• Alpha-2 agonists	

ANTICHOLINERGIC ACTIVITY OF FREQUENTLY USED MEDICATIONS[34]

- **Highly Anticholinergic**
  - Theophylline, prednisolone, cimetidine
- **Moderately Anticholinergic**
  - Furosemide, digoxin, dipyridamole, warfarin, nifedipine, isosorbide, codeine, ranitidine
- **Low Anticholinergic activity**
  - HCTZ/triamterene, captopril
- **Little or no Anticholinergic activity**
  - HCTZ, PPL, nitroglycerin, insulin, ibuprofen, diltiazem, atenolol, timolol, metoprolol

ACTIVE METABOLITES AND ENANTIOMERS[35,36,37]

In the R/S system, based on the specific atoms in the molecule, one configuration is called "rectus" (R- for short) and the other is called "sinister" (S- for short), from the Latin words for right and left. In the D/L system, which is related to how the molecule compares to the chiral molecule glyceraldehyde, one version is called "dextro-" (D- for short) and its mirror image is called "levo-" (L- for short) (from another pair of Latin words for right and left).

Des -Often indicates a demethylated active metabolite of a compound. (Ex: Desvenlafaxine (Pristiq™); Desipramine (Norpramin®); Desloratadine (Clarinex®)

Es or Levo - (Ex: Escitalopram (Lexapro®), Eszopiclone (Lunesta™), Esomeprazole (Nexium®), Levocetirizine (Xyzal®); Levofloxacin (Levaquin®)

Ar or Dextro - (Ex: Arformoterol (Brovana®); Armodafinil (Nuvigil®); Dextroamphetamine (Dexedrine®; Dextrostat®); Dextromethorphan (Robitussin DM®); Dexmethylphenidate (Focalin®)

METABOLITES WHICH ARE MARKETED AS OTHER DRUGS

EFFEXOR® →	PRISTIQ™	LOXITANE® →	ASCENDIN®
Venlafaxine →	desvenlafaxine	Loxapine →	amoxapine
ELAVIL® →	PAMELOR®	MELLARIL® →	SERENTIL®
Amitriptyline →	nortriptyline	Thioridazine →	mesoridazine
TOFRANIL® →	NORPRAMIN®	RISPERDAL® →	INVEGA®
Imipramine →	desipramine	Risperidone →	paliperidone (9-hydroxyrisperidone)

PSYCHIATRIC MEDICATIONS
IMPORTANT SIDE EFFECTS AND MONITORING PARAMETERS

ANTIDEPRESSANTS

Medication/ Class	Important Side Effects	Medical Monitoring Parameters	Important Notes
TCA's/MAOI's	Sedation, Anticholinergic, Cardiac, Sexual dysfunction	EKG	Useful for neuropathic pain
SSRI's (Prozac, Zoloft, Paxil, Luvox, Celexa & Lexapro)	Stimulation, Weight loss, Sedation, Nausea, Vomiting, Diarrhea, Headache, Sweating, Sexual dysfunction	None	Can also treat anxiety, panic attacks, OCD, PTSD, and eating disorders
SNRI's (Effexor & Cymbalta)	Same as SSRI's May increase blood pressure	Blood Pressure Cymbalta - LFTs	Useful for neuropathic pain
Remeron®	Sedation, Weight Gain	Weight, Lipids, etc.	
Wellbutrin®	Anxiety, Stimulation, Dry mouth, Seizures, Insomnia, ↑BP	Watch for seizures	Doses > 200 mg at once ↑ risk for seizures (check on high doses) May ↑ psychosis due to ↑ DA

ANTIPSYCHOTICS

Medication/ Class	Important Side Effects	Medical Monitoring Parameters	Important Notes
TYPICAL ANTIPSYCHOTICS	EPS, Anticholinergic, Cardiac, Weight Gain	EKG, EPS	
ATYPICALS:			Most atypicals are approved for bipolar disorder
Clozaril®	Drowsiness, Dizziness, Weight Gain, Diabetes, Dry mouth, Seizures, Akathisia	WBC, Seizure, Weight, Lipids, Glucose	Higher doses = ↑ seizure risk Must monitor WBCs every week for 1st 6 months
Zyprexa®	Drowsiness, Dizziness, Weight Gain, Diabetes, Akathisia	Weight, Lipids, Glucose	Once daily dosing
Risperdal®, Invega®	Dose-related EPS, Drowsiness, Dizziness, Akathisia	Weight, Lipids, Glucose, EPS, ↑Prolactin	
Seroquel®	Drowsiness, Dizziness, Akathisia	Weight, Lipids, Glucose	BID dosing / XR=evening dose (bipolar depression = QD dosing)
Geodon® or Fanapt®	Drowsiness, Dizziness, QT prolongation, Akathisia	Weight, Lipids, Glucose, EKG	BID dosing
Latuda® or Saphris®	Drowsiness, Dizziness, Akathisia	Weight, Lipids, Glucose, EKG	Watch for allergies with Saphris
Abilify®	Stimulation, GI, headache, Akathisia	Weight, Lipids, Glucose	Should be given QAM (very long half-life), May worsen psychosis if given with another antipsychotic (due to DA agonist properties)

MOOD STABILIZERS

Medication	Important Side Effects	Medical Monitoring Parameters	Important Notes
Lithium®	GI, ↑Thirst, ↑Urination, Mild Tremors, Hypothyroidism	TSH, WBC, renal function	Pregnancy Category D
Valproic Acid /Depakote	GI, Decreased Platelets, ↑LFT's	Platelets, LFT's, Pancreatic enzymes (amylase / lipase)	Teenage girls → polycystic ovarian syndrome Pregnancy Category D
Tegretol®	GI, Dizziness, ↓Na⁺, Diplopia	Na⁺	Pregnancy Category D Enzyme induction / autoinduction
Lamictal®	Rash, GI, Headache	Rash	Must titrate *VERY* slowly to reduce risk of rash Pregnancy Category C

BENZODIAZEPINES

Medication	Important Side Effects	Monitoring Parameters	Important Notes
ALL BENZODIAZEPINES	Drowsiness, Dizziness, Depression, Amnesia, Disinhibition	Watch for abuse	Counsel on withdrawal seizures

9

TRIGGERS OF DEPRESSION[3,4]

NONPSYCHIATRIC MEDICAL CONDITIONS FREQUENTLY ASSOCIATED WITH DEPRESSION	
Cardiovascular Disease	Neurologic disorders (i.e. CVA,
Collagen disorders	Parkinson's, Wilson's Disease)
Endocrine disorders (i.e. hypothyroidism)	Systemic Lupus Erythematosis (SLE)
Infections (i.e. encephalitis, hepatitis, tuberculosis)	Vitamin and mineral deficiencies and
Metabolic disorders	excesses

DRUGS THAT FREQUENTLY CAUSE DEPRESSIVE REACTIONS

Alcohol	Levodopa (Larodopa®, Dopar®)
Amantadine (Symmetrel®)	Methyldopa (Aldomet®)
Beta-blockers	Opiate analgesics
Clonidine (Catapres®)	Oral contraceptives *(Treat with Vitamin B6)*
CNS depressants	Reserpine
Guanethidine (Ismelin®)	Steroids
Hydralazine (Apresoline®)	

TRIGGERS OF ANXIETY[38,39,40,41]

COMMON MEDICAL DISORDERS ASSOCIATED WITH ANXIETY SYMPTOMS	DRUGS ASSOCIATED WITH ANXIETY SYMPTOMS
Cardiovascular/respiratory system	*CNS depressants*
Arrhythmias	Alcohol
Chronic obstructive lung disease	Anxiolytics/sedatives
Hyperdynamic β-adrenergic state	Narcotics (withdrawal from)
Hypertension	**CNS stimulants**
Hyperventilation	*Prescription products*
Mitral valve prolapse (hi correlation to panic)	Albuterol (Proventil®, Ventolin®)
Myocardial infarction	Amphetamines (Dexedrine®)
Angina	Cocaine
Pulmonary embolus	Diethylpropion (Tenuate®)
Endocrine system	Fenfluramine (Pondimin®)
Cushing's disease	Isoproterenol (Isuprel®, Medihaler Iso®)
Hyperthyroidism	Methylphenidate (Ritalin®)
Hypothyroidism	*Non-prescription products*
Hypoglycemia	Caffeine (NoDoz®, Vivarin®)
Pheochromocytoma	Ephedrine (Ephedrine Nasal®)
Gastrointestinal system	Naphazoline (Privine®, Allerest Eye drop®)
Colitis	Oxymetazoline (Afrin®, Dristan®)
Irritable bowel syndrome	Phenylephrine (Neo-Synephrine®, Allerest®)
Peptic ulcer	Phenylpropanolamine (Dexatrim®, Acutrim®)
Ulcerative colitis	Pseudoephedrine (Sudafed®, Novafed®)
Miscellaneous	*Miscellaneous*
Epilepsy	Anticholinergic toxicity
Migraine	Baclofen (Lioresal®)
Pain	Digitalis toxicity
Pernicious anemia	Dapsone
Porphyria	Cycloserine (Seromycin®)
	Quinacrine (Atabrine®)

NON-ADDICTIVE TREATMENTS OF PAIN

NON-MEDICATION:
- Hot or Cold Packs
- Stretching / Limited motion exercises
- Deep Breathing
- Bio-feedback
- Relaxation Tapes
- TENS unit (transcutaneous electrical nerve stimulation)

MEDICATION:
- NSAIDs (Non-Steroidal Anti-Inflammatory Drugs):
  - Motrin®, Advil®, Aleve®, Toradol®, Daypro®, Clinoril®, Celebrex®, Mobic®, many more
- Steroids (anti-inflammatory):
  - Prednisone, Methylprednisone, many more
- Muscle Relaxants (non-addictive):
  - Skelaxin®, Robaxin®, Flexeril®, and others
- Antidepressants – for neuropathic (nerve) pain:
  - Tricyclic Antidepressants (TCAs) – Elavil®, Tofranil®, others
  - Effexor®, Cymbalta®, Serzone®
  - Savella®
- Anticonvulsants - for neuropathic (nerve) pain:
  - Depakote®, Topamax®, Tegretol®, Neurontin®, Lyrica®, others
- Antihistamines:
  - Atarax®, Vistaril®, Benadryl®, others
- Patches and Creams:
  - Catapres TTS® patch, BenGay®, Aspercreme®, Flexall 454®, Arthriticare®, Therapatch®, Ela-max®, Lidoderm® patch, Voltaren® gel, Flector® patch
- Opiate-like pain medicine (non-addictive at normal doses)
  - Ultram®

NON-ADDICTIVE TREATMENTS OF INSOMNIA

NON-MEDICATION:
- Warm Milk
- Toast with Jelly
- Juice or Graham Crackers
  - Think low-protein, high carbohydrate!
- Bananas
- Turkey sandwich (tryptophan)
- Hot Bath or Shower
- Reading a Book or Magazine
- Relaxation Techniques & Tapes
- Deep Breathing Exercises
- Expressing Yourself to Peers or loved ones
  - Maybe by talking it out, you'll be able to fall asleep
- Avoid caffeine, soda, and other stimulating substances late in the day

NON-ADDICTING MEDICATIONS:
- Trazodone (Desyrel®), sedating Tricyclic Antidepressants (e.g.: amitriptyline or doxepin (Silenor®)), ramelteon (Rozerem®), mirtazapine (Remeron®), nefazodone (Serzone®), antihistamines (e.g.: Benadryl®, Unisom®, Atarax® or Vistaril®)
- Zolpidem (Ambien®), zaleplon (Sonata®), or eszopiclone (Lunesta™) at prescribed doses (very large doses can be abused and addictive)

NATURAL PRODUCTS THAT MAY HELP MILD INSOMNIA
- Melatonin
  - Mainly for insomnia associated with jet lag or for shift workers
- Valerian Root, Kava Kava, Lavender, Chamomile

Personality disorders are dysfunctional characteristics of a person's personality. These disorders are incongruent with societal "norms". It is believed that an infant begins forming their personality in the first 2 years of life. Personality disorders have a large environmental component, but may also have a genetic component. People with personality disorders are often unaware of their condition and may feel persecuted by society due to the way they are treated by others. They are divided into Clusters and Types (See DSM-IV TR[1] for detailed information). The three personality clusters are assessed under **Axis II** along with intellectual disabilities. Varying combinations of dysfunction in affectivity, cognition, interpersonal function, and impulse control are observed, based on the type of personality disorder and the cluster into which the disorder is categorized.

> *Cluster A:* The *odd and eccentric cluster* includes the paranoid, schizoid, schizotypal personality d/o.
>
> *Cluster B:* The *dramatic, emotional, erratic cluster* includes the histrionic, narcissistic, antisocial, and borderline personality d/o.
>
> *Cluster C:* The *anxious or fearful cluster* includes avoidant, dependent, and obsessive-compulsive personality d/o.

Cluster A

- Paranoid personality generally manifests within the early adulthood years, and is primarily associated with an intense distrust due to assuming that the motives of others are malicious. Because of the preoccupation with unjustified doubts, a paranoid person may perceive even innocuous interactions as an attack upon his or her character. The result of such an extreme suspicion is that interpersonal relationships are strained the ability to interact becomes stunted.

- Schizoid personality types have a blunted affect that is associated with feelings of detachment. Those with a schizoid personality type may not desire close relationships but rather choose to be solitary. Because they are prone to not show much emotion, others perceive them as having an emotionally cold disposition.

- Those with a schizotypal personality type display a dysfunction in the ability to interact interpersonally due to discomfort. The discomfort does not arise from a negative self-image however, but rather the actual act of having to interact. Schizotypal personality types may also demonstrate cognitive distortions, odd speaking patterns and experience strange perceptual occurrences that influence their behavior.

Cluster B

- Histrionic personality is characterized by a pattern of excessive emotionality and attention seeking. Histrionic types tend to not be happy unless they are the center of attention. In order to gain attention, they may be easily swayed by fads, become overly trusting, and may even interact with others in an inappropriately sexual manner. Displays of emotion are overly dramatic and theatrical, yet are actually superficial and may change immediately.

- Narcissistic personality types are prone to grandiose fantasies with the need for admiration. Generally lacking empathy, narcissists are arrogant and feel a sense of entitlement. They expect others to acknowledge their supposed superiority and will feel overly jealous if others receive praise.

- Those with an antisocial personality demonstrate a pervasive pattern of disregard for and violation of the rights of others. They are extremely impulsive and will show disregard for the safety of others and themselves. Because of this, and that they fail to conform to social norms, they tend to participate in unlawful activities and lack remorse for those whom they have wronged.

- Borderline personality is associated with instability in self-image and interpersonal relationships. Impulsivity that may lead to self-harm, such as substance abuse and promiscuous sex, is typically demonstrated. In many cases, relationships are polarized such that a pattern of extreme idealization and devaluation are expressed. This may lead to feelings of emptiness and frantic efforts to avoid imagined abandonment.

Cluster C

- Avoidant personality types tend to show dysfunction in the ability to interact interpersonally due to discomfort. Unlike the schizotypal personality, however, the discomfort in this case is due to feelings of self-inadequacy. Because of the fear of shame, ridicule, or rejection, those with avoidant personalities may choose to not interact at all. The feeling of inferiority is so pervasive that new activities are rarely attempted and relationships are seldom formed.

- Those with a dependent personality tend to be extremely clingy and display an excessive need to be taken care of. They are prone to experience separation anxiety and will attempt to find another relationship quickly if one ends. It tends to be difficult for them to make every day decisions and they go out of their way to have others take responsibility for major decisions.

- An obsessive-compulsive personality is characterized by an inflexible and rigid strive for perfection. It may be rigid to the point that projects and tasks cannot be completed because they are not perfect enough. The preoccupation with details, rules, lists, and organization can be extremely invasive to the point that it affects interpersonal function.

✶✶*NO MEDICATIONS ARE EFFECTIVE IN TREATING A PERSONALITY DISORDER*✶✶

ATTENTION DEFICIT HYPERACTIVITY DISORDER[42,43,44,45]

- Onset is typically by age 3 and <u>must</u> be by age 7
  - Approx. 9.2% of boys and 2.9% of girls (general prevalence is 6%)
  - Girls generally display inattentive type, while boys exhibit more hyperactive and impulsive type of ADHD.
- Symptoms may persist into adulthood (30-70%)
  - Adult prevalence is 4% by National Comorbidity Survey.
- Clinical Presentation – Inappropriate inattention, Impulsivity, Hyperactivity

- Medications used in ADHD
  - Psychostimulants
    - *February 2006 - An FDA Advisory Panel suggested a Black Box Warning be placed on all stimulant medications, warning of increased risk of CV death and injury*
    - Recent studies find no increased risk of cardiovascular events in children and young to middle-aged adults[46,47]
  - A 10-year study found that stimulants ↑ HR by 4-5 beats per minute, but not BP in children/adolescents[48]
    - o Other studies find no ↑ risk of CV events in children & young to middle-aged adults
  - See page 5 for Black Box Warnings
  - Amphetamines approved for > 3yrs old, methylphenidate approved for > 6 yrs old
  - Approximately 60-75% effective on symptoms
  - MOA: Inhibit the reuptake of dopamine and norepinephrine
    - Also release DA, NE, and 5HT from presynaptic neurons
  - Effects rapidly evident (Response seen in 15-30 minutes and lasts 2-12 hours orally)
  - Side effects:
  - May cause motor or vocal tics and ↑BP
  - May inhibit growth, sleep, and appetite
  - Skin irritation with Daytrana[TM] patch
  - Abdominal pain, weight loss, insomnia, agitation, tachycardia, irritability
    - o Oral doses should be given 30-45 min before meals to reduce anorexia

- Non-stimulants -- Onset of effect may take 3-4 weeks
  - Atomoxetine (Strattera™) – approved for children ≥ 6 years old[49]
    - o MOA: Selective Norepinephrine reuptake inhibitor
    - o Dosing: Start at 0.5mg/kg/day and increase up to 1.2mg/kg/day
      - ▪ Max. dose is 1.4mg/kg/day or 100mg/d
    - o Supplied as 10, 18, 25, 40, and 60 mg capsules
    - o Black Box warning: Potential increase in suicidal ideation/ behavior in pediatric patients
      - ▪ Requires a medication guide be given to patients when dispensed
      - ▪ Contraindicated in patients with seizures or eating disorders

  - Bupropion (Wellbutrin®)[50]
    - o Antidepressant with stimulant-related properties which has been shown effective in both childhood and adult ADHD in several studies over placebo
    - o Average dose in children is 3-6mg/kg/day
    - o Contraindicated in patients with an eating disorder or seizure disorder

  - Alpha2 agonists
    - o Clonidine (Catapres® and KAPVAY™ - an extended release formulation)[51,52]
      - ▪ Decreases hyperactivity and aggressiveness, may be used for sleep
      - ▪ Dosed at 0.004-0.005mg/kg/day (in 0.05mg increments) up to 25mcg/kg/day
      - ▪ Transdermal patch only lasts 5 days in children compared to 7 days in adults

    - o Guanfacine (Tenex®/Intuniv[TM])[53]
      - ▪ Dosing begins at 0.5mg a day (average is 0.5mg twice daily) not to exceed 4mg/d
      - ▪ Intuniv[TM] is dosed QD

  - Antidepressants (TCAs, MAOIs, and SSRIs) are third-line agents
    - o May take weeks to be effective
    - o Caution: cardiac side effects with TCAs and MAOIs

  - Modafinil (Provigil®)[54]
    - o Not FDA approved for ADHD, rather Narcolepsy
      - ▪ Only recommended in adults
      - ▪ Positive results seen with inattention and hyperactivity short-term

13

AMPHETAMINE COMPARISON CHART[55,56,57,58]

Generic Name	Brand Name	Dosing	Dosage Strengths	Duration (hours)	Dosage form
Methyl-phenidate Approved for children ≥ 6 yrs old	Ritalin®	Initially 5-60mg divided Max 2mg/kg/d	5mg, 10mg, 20mg	3-4	Tablets (can cut)
	Methylin CT (chewtab)		2.5mg, 5mg, 10mg	3-4	Tablets (can cut)
	Methylin oral solution		5mg/5ml, 10mg/5ml		Liquid (grape)
	Ritalin SR®		20mg	4-8	Tablets
	Ritalin LA®	20-60mg/d	10mg, 20mg, 30mg, 40mg	8-10	Capsules (sprinkles)
	Metadate ER®		10mg, 20mg	6-8	Tablets
	Metadate CD®	20-60mg QD	10mg, 20mg, 30mg	8-10	Capsules (sprinkles)
	Concerta® See conversions below	18-54mg QD 18-72mg QD (13-17 yr)	18mg, 27mg, 36mg, 54mg	10-12	Tablets
	Daytrana™ (patch)	10-30mg/d	10mg, 15mg, 20mg, 30mg	10-12 (9 hrs on & effects remain 3hrs after removal)	Transdermal patch
Dexmethly-phenidate Approved for children ≥ 6 yrs old	Focalin®	Dose may be adjusted in 2.5-5mg increments to a max of 20mg per day (10mg twice daily).	2.5mg, 5mg, 10mg	4-6	Tablets (can cut)
	Focalin XR®	5-20mg/d	5mg, 10mg, 20mg	6-10	Capsules (sprinkles)
Meth-amphetamine Approved for children ≥ 6 yrs old	Desoxyn®	5-25mg/d	5mg	4-6	Tablets (can cut)
Dextro-amphetamine Approved for children ≥ 3 yrs old	ProCentra® oral solution	2.5-40mg/day	5mg/5ml	4-6	Liquid (bubblegum)
	Dexedrine®		5mg, 10mg		Tablets
	Dextrostat®		5mg, 10mg		Tablets (can cut)
	Dexedrine Spansule®		5mg, 10mg, 15mg	8-12	Capsules (sprinkle)
Mixed Amphetamine salts Approved for children ≥ 3 yrs old	Adderall®	Initially 5mg everyday or twice daily; Titrate 5mg/wk; (Max) 30-60mg/day Based on bioequivalence data, patients taking divided doses of immediate-release ADDERALL, (for example, twice daily), may be switched to ADDERALL XR at the same total daily dose taken once daily.	5mg, 7.5mg, 10mg, 12.5mg, 15mg, 20mg, 30mg	4-6	Tablets (can crush, cut or split)
	Adderall XR®		5mg, 10mg, 15mg, 20mg, 25mg, 30mg	8-12	Capsules (sprinkle)
Lis-dexamfetamine Dimesylate (a prodrug) Approved for children ≥ 6 yrs old	Vyvanse™	Start with 10mg each morning and increase by 20mg each week until good control achieved. MAX DAILY DOSE: 70MG	20mg, 30mg, 40mg, 50mg, 60mg, 70mg	10-12	Capsules (can dissolve in water)

Recommended Dose Conversion from Methylphenidate Regimens to CONCERTA®

5 mg Methylphenidate twice daily or three times daily ≈ 18 mg every morning
10 mg Methylphenidate twice daily or three times daily ≈ 36 mg every morning
15 mg Methylphenidate twice daily or three times daily ≈ 54 mg every morning
20 mg Methylphenidate twice daily or three times daily ≈ 72 mg every morning
Other methylphenidate regimens: Clinical judgment should be used when selecting the starting dose.

14

BIPOLAR MEDICATIONS (Anti-Manics / Mood Stabilizers)[13,14,15,59,60,61,62,63,64,65,66]

- **Lithium (Eskalith®, Lithobid®)**[17]
  - Available as: 150mg, 300mg, 450mg, & 600mg tablets and capsules and 8mEq (300mg)/5ml liquid
  - 95-100% readily absorbed from the GI tract
  - <u>Not</u> protein bound or metabolized / > 95% renally excreted
  - Pre-treatment work-up: SrCr, urinalysis, CBC w/diff, serum electrolytes, glucose, weight, EKG, thyroid function tests (TFTs), history & physical (H & P)
  - Usual starting dose is 300mg BID with food (to reduce GI upset)
  - Serum level range: 0.8 – 1.2 mEq/L (acute phase); 0.4 – 1.0 mEq/L (maintenance phase)
  - Steady state in 5 days of each dosage change; Levels should be drawn 12 hours post dose
  - Early side effects: GI disturbances, lethargy, sedation, headache, ↓ memory & concentration, *polyuria, polydipsia, tremor, dry mouth, leukocytosis (can be beneficial)*
  - Maintenance side effects: fine hand tremor, weight gain, goiter, EKG changes, psoriasis, alopecia, rash, acne, ↓ libido, metallic taste
    - Hypothyroidism
      - Not dose-related, auto-immune related
      - Estimated to be approx. 3% in men and 17% in women from a New Zealand study[67]
      - 5-10X more frequent in women and increased incidence with those > 50 yrs old
        - Usually occurs between 6 – 18 months after starting Lithium
  - Late side effects: nephrogenic diabetes insipidus
  - Meta-analysis found: avg. GFR ↓ by 6.22ml/min, a very small risk of renal failure, odds ratio of developing hypothyroidism of 5.78, ↑ TSH of 4.00iu/ml, ↑ Ca^{++} 0.09mmol/L, ↑ PTH 7.32pg/ml, and an odds ratio of weight gain of 1.89[68]
  - Toxicity side effects: diarrhea, severe nausea and vomiting, coarse hand tremor, hyperreflexia, drowsiness, lethargy, ataxia, blurred vision, dry mouth, large output of dilute urine, confusion, arrhythmias, hypotension, seizures, coma, death
  - Drug interactions: *NSAIDs**, *thiazide diuretics**, *ACEI/ARBS**, neuroleptics, xanthines
    - * = up to 3X ↑Li$^+$ concentrations
  - Contraindications: significant renal, cardiovascular, thyroid disease
    - Pregnancy Category D[69,70,71,72,73,74,75]
      - *(Ebstein's cardiac anomaly)*, caution in breastfeeding, dehydration syndromes
  - Approx. 300mg of lithium carbonate will raise the plasma Li$^+$ concentration by 0.2-0.4 mEq/L in adults
  - Li+(daily dose) = 100.5 + [752.7 x L(ec)] – [3.6 x age] + [7.2 x wt(kg)] – [13.7 x BUN(mg/dl)] where - L(ec) is the expected lithium concentration in mmol/L[76]
  - Li+(daily dose) = 486.8 + (746.83 * level desired) - (10.08 * age) + (5.95 * wt(kg)) + (147.8 * sex) + (92.01 * inpatient) - (74.73 * TCA)[77]
    - sex =1 for male, 0 for female; inpatient = 1 for yes, 0 for no; and TCA use = 1 for yes, 0 for no
    - http://www.russellcottrell.com/md/lithium.shtm - On-line calculator
  - Lithium benefits – highly effective (80-90%)
    - Results of 33 studies revealed a 13 X lower risk of suicide/attempts with long-term Li$^+$ use[78]

- **Valproic acid or divalproex or valproate (Depakote®, Depacon®, Depakote ER®, Stavzor®, Depakene®)**[18]
  - Dosage forms: 125mg/250mg/500mg D.R. tablets, 250mg/500mg ER tablets, 125mg D.R. sprinkle caps, 250mg Regular release caps (Depakene), 100mg/ml injection (Depacon®), 250mg/5ml syrup
  - MOA: inhibits GABA metabolism and ↑ synthesis and release of GABA
  - > 50-90% effective for acute mania and maintenance therapy
  - Baseline assessment: CBC w/diff, LFTs, TFTs, electrolytes, SrCr, BUN, urinalysis, H & P, neurological assessment, EKG
  - Give with food to minimize GI side effects
  - Serum level range: 50-125 µg/ml (acute treatment); 50-100 µg/ml (maintenance)
    - Quick dosing guideline: multiply weight (in lbs.) times 10 (i.e. 150lbs x 10 =1500mg/d)
    - Depakote ER given QD has been shown to produce concentration fluctuations that are 10-20% lower than that of regular divalproex delayed-release tablets given BID, TID, or QID, so must increase dose by 10-20%
      - Draw blood as close to next dose as possible to approximate trough, even if it means going to a lab in the evening[79]
  - Adverse effects: tremors, GI effects, <u>thrombocytopenia</u>, alopecia, rash → up to Steven Johnson's Syndrome
  - **Black Box Warnings:** pancreatitis, teratogenicity, hepatotoxicity
  - Pregnancy Category D[70,71,72,73,74,75]
    - *Neural tube defects / spina bifida*
    - Decreases child's IQ by approx 10 points[80]
    - Increases risk for autism[81]
    - Caution with breastfeeding

- Drug interactions: weak enzyme inhibitor of metabolism, other highly protein bound drugs
- Pooled analysis shows significant response on YMRS (Young Mania Rating Scale) when blood levels are >71.4ug/ml and highest response when levels are >94.1ug/ml[82]
  - o Tolerability was similar at all dosages

- **Carbamazepine (CBZ) (Tegretol®, Tegretol XR®, Equetro™, Epitol®, Carbatrol®)**[19]
  - Dosage forms: 100mg chew tabs, 200mg tablet, 100mg/200mg/400mg ER tablets (Tegretol XR), 100mg/200mg/300mg ER capsules (Carbatrol/Equetro), 100mg/5ml suspension
  - MOA: structure similar to TCAs; ↓ kindling (rapid cycling), ↓ DA and GABA turnover
  - 60% effective for acute mania; 60-75% effective for prophylaxis
  - Baseline assessment: same as Depakote®
  - Draw levels in 1-2 weeks, then biweekly for 2 months, then every 2-4 months if necessary
  - Adverse effects: neurotoxicity, nystagmus, diplopia, GI upset, dry mouth, rash → Steven Johnson's Syndrome, hematological changes, hyponatremia / SIADH, hepatic changes
  - Caution with breastfeeding; Pregnancy Category D
    - o Must counsel patients about birth control pills not being effective due to enzyme induction
  - Drug interactions: enzyme inducer of all drugs metabolized by liver; enzyme inhibitors ↑CBZ levels (cimetidine, fluoxetine); protein bound drugs
  - Auto-inducer of its own metabolism – should re-check CBZ levels in 5 weeks because levels may go down and dose may have to be increased

- **Lamotrigine (Lamictal®)**[83]
  - FDA approved for maintenance of Bipolar I (not for acute treatment)
  - Concerns: Rash in 0.08-0.3% of adults (higher in children) (must be titrated slowly to avoid rash)
  - Side effects: Nausea, insomnia, headache, somnolence, back/abdominal pain, fatigue, rhinitis
  - Dosing depends on other drugs being given
    - o Use a lower dose of lamotrigine when given with a glucuronidation inhibitor (ie. valproate)
    - o Use a higher dose of lamotrigine when given with a glucuronidation inducer
  - Change dose every 1-2 weeks / start with 25mg + QD depending on other drugs being used
  - Pregnancy Category C
  - Patients on birth control pills should take it all month long (no off weeks) to keep levels consistent
    - o Combined oral contraceptives can ↓ lamotrigine levels by 25-50%[84]

	With Valproic acid	As monotherapy	With an EIAED*
Weeks 1&2	25mg QOD or 12.5mg QD	25mg QD	50mg QD
Weeks 3&4	25mg QD	25mg BID or 50mg QD	50mg BID
Weekly dose ↑ thereafter	25mg	25 or 50mg	50-100mg
Average maintenance dose	100-200mg QD (or ÷ BID)	200-400mg QD or ÷ BID	300-500mg (÷ BID)
*EIAED = Enzyme-inducing Anti-epileptic Drug, such as: carbamazepine, phenytoin, phenobarbital, primidone, rifampin, estrogen-containing oral contraceptives			

- **Olanzapine [OLZ] and fluoxetine [FLX] HCl capsules (Symbyax®)**[85]
  - FDA approved for bipolar depression and Treatment Resistant Depression
  - Available in 3/25mg, 6/25mg, 6/50mg, 12/25mg, and 12/50mg capsules [OLZ/FLX]
  - Side effects: Drowsiness, weight gain, increased appetite, feeling weak, swelling, tremor, sore throat and difficulty concentrating

- **Quetiapine (Seroquel®)**[86]
  - FDA approved as monotherapy for bipolar depression
  - Average dose in study responders was approximately 300mg/d

- **Oxcarbazepine (Trileptal®)**[87]
  - Not FDA approved for bipolar disorder
  - Can be considered as a third line option when all other options have failed
  - Randomized controlled trials have had mixed results in adults and in children found no significant improvement in mania symptoms as compared to placebo[88]

16

MAJOR DEPRESSION AND ANTIDEPRESSANTS[89,90,91,92,93,94,95,96,97]

♦ Depressive symptoms must be present for > 2 weeks to diagnose, along with $\geq$4 SIGECAPS (acronym for symptoms)[1]
♦ Recurrence rates of major depression:[3,98,99]

	After 1 year	After 2 years	After 5 years
After 1st episode	25%	42%	60%
After 2nd episode	41%	59%	74%

♦ Length of antidepressant treatment[2]
  ♦ 1st time depressed → 6 months to 1 year
  ♦ 2nd time depressed → 2 years (have 70% chance of relapse)
  ♦ 3 or more times depressed → lifetime therapy
    o Have >90% chance of relapse
♦ 60-70% response rate, remission rates are lower ≈ 30-40%
♦ Can take 2-6 weeks to work (sometimes even up to 12 weeks)
  ♦ *Always titrate up for best tolerability to side effects*
♦ All antidepressants lower seizure threshold!!
  ♦ Highest risk with bupropion, amoxapine, and maprotiline (BAM)
♦ Non-addictive
♦ Antidepressant Discontinuation Syndrome (ADS)[100,101,102,103]
  ♦ Antidepressant withdrawal associated with an antidepressant's side effects
  ♦ Occurs mostly with short half-life antidepressants
  ♦ Tricyclics withdrawal may include cholinergic "rebound" such as abdominal cramping, diarrhea, Parkinsonism and other problems with movement
  ♦ Characterized by the "FINISH" syndrome:
    • *F*lu-like symptoms
    • *I*nsomnia
    • *N*ausea
    • *I*mbalance
    • *S*ensory disturbances
    • *H*yperarousal (anxiety/agitation)

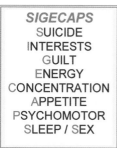

SIGECAPS
SUICIDE
INTERESTS
GUILT
ENERGY
CONCENTRATION
APPETITE
PSYCHOMOTOR
SLEEP / SEX

HETEROCYCLIC / TCA AGENTS (SEE CHART ON PAGE 3)
♦ MOA: 5HT/NE reuptake inhibitor
♦ Evaluate suicide potential because toxic doses (750-1500mg) can kill!!
♦ Pregnancy category B or C
♦ Adverse reactions: drowsiness, CNS stimulation (2° amines), toxic psychosis
  ♦ Anticholinergic effects (dry mouth, constipation, tachycardia etc.)
  ♦ Autonomic side effects (nasal congestion, tremors, sexual dysfunction)
  ♦ Cardiac side effects (arrhythmias, Q-T interval prolongation, hypotension/orthostasis)
  ♦ Weight gain, seizures, allergic reactions, agranulocytosis (rare)

MONOAMINE OXIDASE INHIBITORS (SEE CHART ON PAGE 3)
♦ MOA: irreversibly inhibit MAO with a 2 week duration of effect
♦ Adverse reactions: postural hypotension, hepatic complications, anticholinergic effects (less than TCAs), sedation (most with phenelzine), stimulation (most with tranylcypromine), hypertensive crisis (tyramine-containing foods, sympathomimetic-containing drugs), sexual dysfunction
♦ *SIGNIFICANT* drug-drug and food-drug interactions – USE THESE DRUGS WITH CAUTION!!!
♦ Emsam® (selegiline patch) – no dietary restrictions necessary at 6 mg/d dose

SELECTIVE SEROTONIN REUPTAKE INHIBITORS (SSRIs)
♦ *Adverse reactions*: weight loss, anorexia, anxiety, insomnia, headache, sweating, nausea, diarrhea, sexual dysfunction (very common, but under-reported by patients)

  ♦ Fluoxetine (Prozac®, Sarafem®)[104]
    ♦ Active metabolite- norfluoxetine
      ♦ $T_{1/2}$ = 4-16 days (VERY LONG!!!) – including active metabolite
      ♦ may be good for non-compliant patients
    ♦ 95% protein bound
    ♦ Potent inhibitor of P450-2D6
    ♦ Dosing: 10-80 mg/d usually given in the AM (to reduce insomnia)
    ♦ New generic 60mg scored tablet available (Edgemont Pharmaceuticals)
    ♦ Drug interactions: MAOIs or Tryptophan (serotonin syndrome), other highly protein bound drugs, other drugs metabolized by P450-2D6

- Sertraline (Zoloft®)[105]
  - Active metabolite- desmethylsertraline
  - ≥ 97% protein bound
  - Minor inhibitor of P450-2D6 and P450-3A4 (not very significant)
  - Dosing: 25-200 mg/d usually given in the AM (to reduce insomnia)
  - Slightly more GI side effects than Prozac
- Paroxetine (Paxil®/Paxil CR®/Pexeva®)[106]
  - NO active metabolites
  - 95% protein bound
  - P450-2D6 enzyme inhibitor > Prozac
  - Dosing: 10-60 mg/d usually given at HS
  - Most sedating, anticholinergic, and most likely to cause long-term weight gain of the SSRIs
  - Pregnancy Category D!!![107]
    - o Not good for breastfeeding
  - FDA has issued a warning against its use in children due to increased emotional lability!!!
- Fluvoxamine (Luvox®/Luvox CR®)[108]
  - Metabolized by P450-1A2 and P450-3A4 (potent inhibitor) > 9 metabolites (most inactive)
  - 80% protein bound
  - ↓ clearance with hepatic impairment
  - Should be given with food to decrease nausea
  - Usually dosed in the PM (AM if insomnia occurs) or BID - Luvox CR® is QD
  - Drug interactions: MAOIs, inhibits P450-1A2 and P450-3A4, propranolol and metoprolol (bradycardia/hypotension), triazolam and alprazolam (↑ levels), digoxin and warfarin (↑ levels), smoking ↑ clearance by 25%, lithium (seizures), tryptophan (vomiting)
- Citalopram (Celexa®)[109]
  - Metabolized by P450-3A4 and P450-2C19
  - 80% protein bound
  - Drug interactions with QT-prolonging drugs (absolute contraindication!)
  - Less adverse reactions than other SSRIs
  - Adult Dosing: 10-40 mg/d (clinical trials showed 60mg no more effective than 40mg)
    - o 60mg dose ↑ QTc by about 18.5msec (mostly due to R-enantiomer)
    - o http://www.fda.gov/Drugs/DrugSafety/ucm269086.htm
  - Elderly (over 60 y.o.) or pts receiving potent CYP2C9 Inhibitors: max dose of 20mg/d
- Escitalopram (Lexapro®)[110]
  - S-optical isomer (enantiomer) of citalopram
  - 2-4 times as potent as citalopram
  - Little or no drug interactions
  - Dosing: 5-20 mg/d (max dose for geriatric patients is 10 mg/day)

SSRI INDICATIONS (ASIDE FROM ADULT DEPRESSION)

	Pediatric Depression	Pediatric OCD*	Adult OCD	Bulimia Nervosa	PTSD **	PMDD ***	GAD ****	Social Anxiety Disorder	Panic Disorder
Prozac	X		X	X		X			X
Zoloft		X	X		X	X		X	X
Paxil	(FDA WARNING)		X		X	Paxil CR	X	X	X
Luvox		X	X					Luvox CR	
Celexa									
Lexapro	X						X		

*OCD = Obsessive-Compulsive Disorder   **PTSD = Post-traumatic Stress Disorder
***PMDD = Premenstrual Dysphoric Disorder   ****GAD = Generalized Anxiety Disorder

APPROXIMATE DOSE EQUIVALENTS OF ANTIDEPRESSANTS

Drug	Dose	T ½ hrs	CYP* substrate	CYP* inhibitor
Fluoxetine	20mg	>4-6 days	2D6 partially	POTENT 2D6 Inhibitor
Paroxetine	20mg	21 hrs	2D6, 3A4 rarely	POTENT 2D6 inhibitor
Citalopram	20mg	35 hrs	3A4, 2C19	Mild 2D6
Escitalopram	10mg	27-32 hrs	3A4, 2C19 Mild 2D6	
Sertraline	50-75mg	24 hrs	2B6/D6, 2C9/19,3A4	DOSES >200mg all CYP
Venlafaxine	75mg	5 & 11 hrs	2D6	Mild 2D6
Fluvoxamine	100mg	22-30 hrs	------	2C9/19, 3A4, 1A2
Duloxetine	30mg	12.5-19.1 hrs	2D6	Mild 2D6
Desvenlafaxine	50mg	11 hrs	------	------

*CYP is the Cytochrome P450 enzyme system

OTHER ANTIDEPRESSANTS

- **Bupropion (Zyban® / Wellbutrin®, SR, XL / Aplenzin® - HBr salt / Forfivo™ XL / Budeprion®)**[50]
  - A derivative of the weight loss medication *diethylpropion* (Tenuate®)
  - MOA: weak DA and NE reuptake inhibitor (??? truly unknown)
  - Usually dosed in the AM and mid afternoon (not too late because of insomnia)
  - Not to exceed 450 mg/d (150mg TID regular release) or XL and 400 mg/d SR due to seizure risk
  - Adverse reactions: nausea, vomiting, constipation, dry mouth, headache, nervousness, dermatologic reactions, little sexual dysfunction
  - Contraindicated in those with seizures or eating disorders, or abruptly discontinuing EtOH or BZDs
  - May be as effective as Ritalin® for ADD/ADHD in adults
  - Lesser risk of inducing mania in bipolar patients compared to SSRIs
  - Good choice for depressed smokers wanting to quit (Zyban® is indicated in smoking cessation)
  - Aplenzin®: 174mg, 348mg, and 522mg extended-release tablets

- **Duloxetine (Cymbalta®)**[111]
  - Also approved for chronic musculoskeletal pain, GAD, Fibromyalgia, and Diabetic nerve pain
  - A serotonin and norepinephrine reuptake inhibitor
  - >90% plasma protein binding
  - Elimination half-life of 12 hours
  - Metabolized by P450-1A2 and 2D6 (inhibitor)
  - Dosing: Begin with 20mg QD, Max dose is 120mg a day (QD or divided BID)
  - Availability: 20mg, 30mg, and 60mg enteric coated capsules
  - Contraindications: Narrow-angle glaucoma
  - Side effects: Anticholinergic, drowsiness, nausea, ↓ appetite, sweating, sexual dysfunction
    - Watch for rare hepatotoxicity

- **Venlafaxine (Effexor®)**[112]
  - Also approved for GAD, Panic disorder (with/without agoraphobia) and social phobia
  - MOA: 5HT > NE and weak DA reuptake inhibitor
  - 27% protein bound
  - Metabolized by P450-2D6 to 3 active metabolites
  - Adverse reactions similar to SSRIs (More nausea / may ↑ BP)
    - Give with food to ↓ nausea
    - Caution in patients with uncontrolled BP
  - Dosing: 75-375 mg/d
    - Maximum of 225mg QD for XR and 375mg divided BID-TID for RR
    - RR formulation = tablets; XR formulation = capsules
  - May be beneficial to those with neuropathic pain syndromes
  - Drug interactions: drugs that inhibit P450-2D6 ↑ venlafaxine levels, MAOIs

- **Desvenlafaxine (Pristiq™)**[113]
  - MOA: Major metabolite of venlafaxine in an extended-release tablet
  - Dosing: 50mg QD up to a max of 100mg QD (no benefit in studies though)
  - Half-life of 11 hours

- **Trazodone (Desyrel® / Oleptro™)**[114,115]
  - MOA: less potent SSRI, 5HT agonist, 5HT2A/2C antagonist (???)
  - Caution: Its active metabolite (mCPP) can trigger a migraine headache when mCPP's vasoconstricting properties wear off (usually the morning after taking it)
  - Dosing: 25-400 mg/d given at HS (used for sleep) or divided
    - Up to 600mg/d can be used in hospitalized patients
  - 92% protein bound
  - Adverse reactions: priapism (very rare), drowsiness, orthostasis, anticholinergic effects
  - Oleptro™ is available in 150mg and 300mg scored extended-release tablets
    - Contramid® technology, so tablets can be broken in half

- **Nefazodone (Serzone®)**[116] – Brand name withdrawn from US market due to rare liver failure
  - MOA: NE and 5HT reuptake inhibitor and 5HT2 blocker
    - 5HT$_2$ blockade = ↓ anxiety and ↓ sexual dysfunction
  - Food delays and decreases absorption by 20%
  - Active metabolite can cause migraine headache, as with trazodone
  - > 99% protein bound
  - Metabolized by P450-3A4 (potent inhibitor) to 2 active metabolites
  - Dosing: 50-600 mg/d divided BID
  - Adverse reactions: anticholinergic effects, nausea, drowsiness, weakness, orthostasis
  - Drug interactions:
    - Triazolam, alprazolam, theophylline levels ↑, MAOIs, protein bound drugs

- **Vilazodone (Viibryd™)**[117] - Distributed by Trovis Pharmaceuticals LLC
  - MOA - SSRI + 5HT1a receptor partial agonist (like buspirone)
  - Available in 10mg, 20mg, and 40mg tablets
  - Dosing is 10mg/d x7d, then 20mg/d x7d, then 40mg/d thereafter (WITH FOOD)
    - Food ↑ AUC X2 (ie. twice as much drug is absorbed by the body)
    - 30 day starter kits are available
  - Side effects: diarrhea (28%), nausea (23%), vomiting (5%), insomnia (6%), sexual dysfunction
    - No significant effects on weight or BP
  - Metabolized by Cytochrome P450-3A4 mostly (minor by P450-2C19 and P450-2D6)
    - Any inhibitors or inducers of P450-3A4 will affect Vilazodone blood levels
  - May inhibit CYP2C8 substrates
  - Half-life is 25 hours
  - 96-99% protein bound
  - Pregnancy Category C

- **Mirtazapine (Remeron® / SolTabs®)**[118]
  - MOA: alpha2 antagonist, blocks post-synaptic 5HT2 and 5HT3 receptors, high H1 blockade, weak antagonist of muscarinic and alpha1 receptors
    - 5HT₃ blockade = anti-emetic effects
    - 5HT₂ blockade = ↓ anxiety and ✓ *sexual dysfunction*
  - 85% protein bound
  - Metabolized by P450-2D6, 1A2, 3A4
  - Dosing: 15-45 mg/d usually given at HS
  - Most common adverse reactions: somnolence, ↑ appetite, weight gain, dizziness
  - Has been shown in studies to work a little faster than other antidepressants, but exact details remain unknown
  - Drug interactions: MAOIs, maybe clonidine because of opposing mechanism (??)

ANTIDEPRESSANTS WITH LOWEST RISK OF SEXUAL DYSFUNCTION
- **Wellbutrin®, Remeron®, and Serzone®**

ANTIDEPRESSANTS' MECHANISM OF ACTION EXPLAINED

Once antidepressants (SSRI, SNRI, TCA, etc) are initiated, there is an increase in neurotransmission, the postsynaptic receptors begin to down-regulate and this correlates with antidepressant response. As you can see in the above picture down-regulation of postsynaptic receptors takes time after medication is initiated.

When initiating antidepressants it is like putting fertilizer on grass or plants. Example: If you put fertilizer down on the grass or plant, it takes several weeks for the grass or plant to turn green. The fertilizer needs to be absorbed and gradually make changes. This is the similar case when you begin & continue taking antidepressant medication. It can take several weeks (2-6 weeks) for optimal pharmacologic response to occur as medication needs to cause postsynaptic downregulation or in other layman's terms "get into the roots of the system".

**IV Ketamine, in small doses, is currently being studied in controlled settings for rapid onset/relief of depressive symptoms and for treatment resistant depression. **

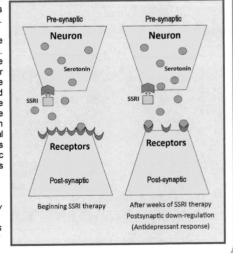

Beginning SSRI therapy

After weeks of SSRI therapy
Postsynaptic down-regulation
(Antidepressant response)

COMMON ANTIDEPRESSANT SIDE EFFECTS

TRICYCLIC ANTIDEPRESSANTS:

▶ ANTICHOLINERGIC SIDE EFFECTS
- Blurred vision
- Constipation
- Dry mouth
- Tachycardia
- Urinary retention
- Decreased memory
- Delirium
- Cholinergic rebound upon abrupt withdrawal

▶ CNS EFFECTS:
- Drowsiness (very common)
- Stimulation (more with 2° amines)
- Toxic Psychosis (Anticholinergic effect)

▶ AUTONOMIC SIDE EFFECTS
- Nasal congestion
- Tremors
- Sexual dysfunction (less than with SSRIs)

▶ SEIZURES
- Highest with Amoxapine and Maprotiline
- All antidepressants lower seizure threshold!!!

▶ OTHER:
- Weight gain
- Allergic rxn's
  - Rash, urticaria, photosensitivity, fever
- Agranulocytosis (rare)
- Hepatic obstructive jaundice (very rare)
- Endocrinologic (i.e. SIADH)
- Caution in pregnancy and breastfeeding!

▶ CARDIAC SIDE EFFECTS
- Heart Block - 1° or 2° is contraindicated
- Arrhythmias - prolong Q-T interval
- Hypotension / orthostasis
- Tachycardia (Direct, anticholinergic, and reflex)

MONOAMINE OXIDASE INHIBITORS:
- Postural hypotension
- Hepatic complications hydrazine > non-hydrazine
- Anticholinergic (less than TCAs)
- Sedation (most with phenelzine)
- Stimulation (most with tranylcypromine)
- Sexual dysfunction
- **Hypertensive crisis:**
  - *Tyramine*-containing foods

SELECTIVE SEROTONIN REUPTAKE INHIBITORS:
- Sexual dysfunction
- Anxiety
- Insomnia
- Weight loss / wt. gain (long-term)
- Headache
- Sweating
- Nausea
- Diarrhea
- Hyponatremia
- Rare abnormal bleeding

SEROTONIN NOREPINEPHRINE REUPTAKE INHIBITORS:
- Similar to SSRIs
- Somnolence (drowsiness)
- Dry mouth
- Dizziness
- Hypertension
- Orthostatic hypotension

MIRTAZAPINE (REMERON®):
- Somnolence
- Increased appetite with weight gain
- Dizziness

BUPROPION (WELLBUTRIN®)
- Anxiety
- Weight loss
- Seizures
- Insomnia
- Hypertension

SEROTONIN SYNDROME

Serotonin syndrome is characterized by rapid development of hyperthermia, hypertension, myoclonus (involuntary muscle twitching), rigidity, autonomic instability, mental status changes (e.g., delirium or coma), and in rare cases, death.

First-line treatment of serotonin syndrome is to withdraw the offending drugs and to provide supportive care. On the basis of case reports, moderate to severe cases of serotonin syndrome may be treated with cyproheptadine, an antihistamine and a serotonin-receptor antagonist.[119] Cyproheptadine: Give 12mg po, then +/- 2mg Q2h until improvement seen.

Hunter Serotonin Toxicity Criteria[120]	Sternbach Criteria for Serotonin Syndrome[121]
In the presence of a serotonergic agent and one of the following symptoms: 1. Spontaneous clonus 2. Inducible clonus and agitation or diaphoresis 3. Ocular myoclonus and agitation or diaphoresis 4. Ocular myoclonus or inducible clonus 5. Tremor and hyperreflexia or hypertonia 6. Temperature >38°C and ocular myoclonus or inducible clonus	1. Recent addition or increase in a known serotonergic agent 2. Absence of other possible etiologies (eg., infection, substance abuse, withdrawal, etc) 3. No recent addition or increase of a neuroleptic agent 4. At least 3 of the following symptoms: Mental status changes (confusion, hypomania), agitation, myoclonus, hyperreflexia, diaphoresis, shivering, tremor, diarrhea, incoordination, or fever

Clinical Presentation:

➢ <u>Cognitive effects</u>: mental confusion, hypomania, hallucinations, agitation, headache, coma
➢ <u>Autonomic effects</u>: shivering, sweating, hyperthermia, hypertension, tachycardia, nausea, diarrhea
➢ <u>Somatic effects</u>: myoclonus, hyperreflexia, clonus, tremor

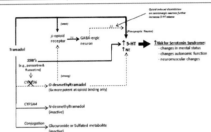

Reprinted with permission from Pharmacology Weekly

<u>Tramadol</u>: SSRIs such as fluoxetine and paroxetine may inhibit the formation of the active M1 metabolite of tramadol by inhibiting CYP2D6. The inhibition of this metabolite may decrease the analgesic effectiveness of tramadol but increase the level of the parent compound, which has more serotonergic activity than the metabolite.

Serotonin Receptor Agonists and Antagonists:

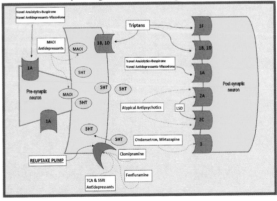

Serotonin Receptors	Consequence of Serotonin Stimulation
5HT1	Antidepressant Anxiolytic
5HT2	Anxiety Agitation Insomnia Sexual dysfunction
5HT 3	GI distress Nausea Diarrhea Headache

▲ The misconception that 5-HT1a receptors can cause serious SS is still widely perpetuated
▲ Quality evidence reveals that activation of the 5-HT2a receptor is required for SS.[122,123,124,125,126,127]
▲ *SS is unlikely to evolve from an SSRI + triptans based upon literature and mechanism involved*
▲ Of the 29 cases used for the basis of the FDA alert, only 10 cases actually met the Sternbach Criteria for diagnosing serotonin syndrome, and none met the Hunter Criteria.
▲ Cautious use of SSRIs with other compounds that are serotonergic is advised. The likelihood of SS to evolve from SSRI & triptans is unlikely based upon literature and mechanism involved. There is possibility of SS with SSRIs and cyclobenzaprine, as it's structurally similar to tricyclic antidepressants.[128] The incidence is unlikely, but caution is still advised as there are a handful of case reports. While SSRIs and tramadol are commonly prescribed concomitantly—it is advised to exercise caution—especially with CYP-2D6 inhibitors (paroxetine & fluoxetine).

DSM-IV TR ANXIETY DISORDERS[1]
* Generalized Anxiety Disorder (GAD)
* Social and Simple Phobias
* Obsessive-Compulsive Disorder (OCD)
* Panic Disorder
* Post-Traumatic Stress Disorder (PTSD)

Buspirone (Buspar®)[12]
* MOA- 5HT1a partial agonist
* Onset of action 2-4 weeks → Not for prn therapy
* Metabolized by P450-2D6
* Start at 5mg po TID and ↑ by 5mg/day every 2-3 days as tolerated
* Avg. dose: 20-30 mg/d divided; anxiolytic effects: 10-60 mg/d
* Adverse reactions: nausea, dysphoria, headache, weakness, dizziness, nervousness
* Drug interactions: MAOIs, fluoxetine & paroxetine ↑ buspirone levels

BENZODIAZEPINES
* Drugs of choice for short-term prn tx of Generalized Anxiety Disorder (GAD)
* All BZDs are similar in sedative, hypnotic, anxiolytic, muscle relaxation, and anticonvulsant activity
* Absorption determines onset of action
    * Rapid: diazepam, clorazepate, alprazolam (15-60 minutes)
    * Intermediate: chlordiazepoxide, lorazepam
    * Slow: prazepam, oxazepam, temazepam, clonazepam
* Most BZDs are metabolized to active metabolites except lorazepam, oxazepam, temazepam (LOT)
    * These agents are ideal for elderly patients as no extensive metabolism (Phase II conjugation)
* Adverse reactions: sedation, fatigue, depression, dizziness, ataxia, paradoxical excitement, agitation, confusion, disorientation, anterograde amnesia, respiratory depression, disinhibition
* Drug interactions: CNS depressants, alcohol, cimetidine (except LOT); nefazodone and fluvoxamine drastically ↑ alprazolam/triazolam levels
* Due to abuse potential, dependence, withdrawal and tolerance use should not exceed 4 months
    * Although, physical dependence can occur in as little as 2 weeks
* Seizures are possible with acute withdrawal (must taper!!)
* Long-term benzodiazepine use is associated with high socioeconomic costs[130]
* Use is associated with an increased risk of, and mortality from Community Acquired Pneumonia[131]

PTSD[1]

An individual is exposed to a traumatic event in which both were present:
(1) Person (experienced, witnessed, or confronted) with an event that involved actual or threatened death, serious injury or physical integrity to self or others.
(2) The individual's response involved intense fear, helplessness or horror.

Re-experiencing (One or more)	Avoidance (Three or more)	Hyperarousal (Two or more)
• Intrusive Memories (IMs) • Nightmares (NMs) • Feel as if traumatic event recurring • Intense psychological distress at exposure to internal or external cues symbolizing/resembling traumatic event • Intense psychological distress at exposure to internal/external cues symbolizing/resembling traumatic event • Physiologic reactivity on exposure to internal/external cues symbolizing/resembling traumatic event.	• Thoughts/feelings/conversations associated with trauma • Activities, places, people that arouse recollections of the trauma • Inability to recall an important aspect of trauma • Markedly diminished interest in activities • Feeling of detachment/ estrangement from others • Restricted range of affect • Sense of foreshortened future	• Difficulties concentrating • Exaggerated startle response • Hypervigilance • Irritability/Anger outbursts • Difficulties sleeping

Pharmacologic Tx: only **Paroxetine & Sertraline** are FDA approved meds though other SSRIs are considered beneficial.
SNRIs-beneficial and first line
TCAs-beneficial and second line
SGAs-suggested in psychotic symptoms
Alpha 2 Agonists-Clonidine
Alpha 1 Blockers-Prazosin (cross BBB)
Others: Mirtazapine, Nefazodone, Phenelzine, Anti-epileptic drugs (mood stabilizers) have questionable benefits.
Avoid Yohimbine (Alpha 2 Antagonist)-readily crosses BBB and can produce CNS effects (IMs, FBs, NMs, agitation, etc)

Most Anxiety Disorders Respond Very Well to Psychotherapy and/or Antidepressants!
BENZODIAZEPINES ARE NOT RECOMMENDED FOR LONG-TERM USE!!!

COMPARISON OF COMMON BENZODIAZEPINES[132-144]

Drug	Relative Potency	Peak Blood Level -oral (hours)	Half-life (hours)	Equivalent Dose (mg)	Dosage range (mg/d)	Notes
Triazolam (Halcion)	HIGH	1 - 2	1.5 - 5	0.25	0.125 - 0.5	Cytochrome P450 3A4 substrate
Clonazepam (Klonopin)	HIGH	1 - 4	19 - 60	0.25	0.25 - 20	Cytochrome P450 3A4 substrate
Alprazolam (Xanax)	HIGH	1 - 2	9 - 20	0.5	0.25 - 10	Cytochrome P450 3A4 substrate
Lorazepam (Ativan)	HIGH	1 - 4	8 - 24	1	0.5 - 10	Conjugated, not metabolized
Estazolam (ProSom)	HIGH	1 - 2	10 - 24	?	0.5 - 2	Cytochrome P450 3A4 substrate
Diazepam (Valium)	MEDIUM	1 - 2	100	5	2 - 40	Cytochrome P450 3A4 substrate
Clorazepate (Tranxene)	MEDIUM	0.5 - 2	100	7.5 - 10	3.75 - 90	Pro-drug
Flurazepam (Dalmane)	MEDIUM	0.5 - 1	40 - 250	15 - 30	15 - 60	Cytochrome P450 3A4 substrate
Oxazepam (Serax)	LOW	1 - 4	6 - 25	15	10 - 120	Conjugated, not metabolized
Chlordiazepoxide (Librium)	LOW	1 - 4	100	10 - 25	5 - 400	
Temazepam (Restoril)	LOW	2 - 3	8 - 25	10 - 30	15 - 60	Conjugated, not metabolized

ANTIPSYCHOTICS (NEUROLEPTICS / MAJOR TRANQUILIZERS)[7,145-148]

- ◆ DIFFERENTIAL PSYCHOTIC DISORDERS:
  - ◆ **Brief Psychotic Disorder** – Psychosis that lasts at least 1 day and remits in < 30 days
  - ◆ **Schizophreniform Disorder** – Psychosis that lasts 1 to 6 months
  - ◆ **Schizophrenia** – Psychosis that persists > 6 months
  - ◆ **Schizoaffective Disorder** – a mood episode (eg. Bipolar) and Schizophrenia co-occur

---

TARGET SYMPTOMS OF SCHIZOPHRENIA: (POSITIVE & NEGATIVE)

POSITIVE SYMPTOMS: things that happen that should not happen

delusions	grandiosity	**Typical & Atypical**
conceptual disorganization	hostility	Neuroleptics
excitement	hallucinations	treat these symptoms
suspiciousness / persecution		

NEGATIVE SYMPTOMS: things that should happen and do not happen

difficulty in abstract thinking	blunted mood	
lack of spontaneity	emotional withdrawal	**Atypical** Neuroleptics
flow of conversation	poor rapport	treat these symptoms
apathetic social withdrawal	stereotyped thinking	

- ▶ Cognitive symptoms / Executive function (learning from one's mistakes)
  - • Only **Atypical** Antipsychotics treat these symptoms

- ◆ ANTIPSYCHOTIC EFFECTIVENESS
  - ◆ A drug must block between 65 and 78% of D2 receptors in the striatum to reduce psychosis
    - o 2mg to 5mg a day of haloperidol achieves maximal blockade in this range
    - o *CNS Drugs* 2001:15(9):671-8.[149,150,151,152,153]
  - ◆ Some atypical antipsychotics do not exceed 78% due to loose D2 binding
    - o Result is little or no EPS
  - ◆ With medication, relapse rate in Schizophrenia is < 30% per year
  - ◆ <u>Without</u> medication, relapse rate is 60-70% in 1 year, 90% in 2 years

- ◆ SIDE EFFECTS OF TYPICAL ANTIPSYCHOTICS (ALSO CALLED 1ST GENERATION)
  - ◆ Related to the potency of the drug on D2 blockade (see RELATIVE POTENCIES on next page)
  - ◆ Low potency drugs are highest in anticholinergic, antihistaminic, alpha-1 blockade
    (ie. orthostatic hypotension), but are low in EPS
  - ◆ High potency drugs are high in EPS, but low in anticholinergic and other side effects
  - ◆ Extrapyramidal Side Effects (EPS)
    - o **Acute dystonias** *(an emergency situation)* - sudden onset of muscle contraction
    - o **Pseudoparkinsonism** – resembles Parkinson's Disease
    - o **Akathisias** *(restlessness)*
    - o **Tardive dyskinesia** – Involuntary movements of the face, mouth, arms, legs
    - o Happens because of an imbalance between dopamine and acetylcholine (Ach)
    - o Treatment of EPS:
      - ▪ Benztropine (Cogentin®) 1-8 mg/d divided BID
      - ▪ Trihexyphenidyl (Artane®) 2-15 mg/d divided TID
      - ▪ Biperiden (Akineton®) 2-8 mg/d
      - ▪ Diphenhydramine (Benadryl®) 50-400 mg/d
      - ▪ Amantadine 100-300 mg/d (useful for tremors) divided TID
      - ▪ Lorazepam or diazepam for acute treatment
      - ▪ Propranolol 20-60 mg/d or more (drug of choice for akathisia)

    DA↓ Ach↑

  - • Other potential side effects with Typical antipsychotics
    - o Cardiovascular
      - ▲ Arrhythmias
      - ▲ Tachycardia from Vagal inhibition, Reflex tachycardia, and Quinidine-like effects
    - o Photophobia / Photosensitivity
    - o Dermatological rash and discolorations (Blue-gray skin discoloration)
    - o Hepatologic issues (Up to 50% have transiently ↑ed LFTs)
    - o Hematologic (blood dyscrasias including agranulocytosis)
    - o Hormonal
      - ▲ ↑ prolactin, amenorrhea, gynecomastia
      - ▲ Sexual Dysfunction in 25-60% of patients
    - o Thermoregulation difficulties
    - o Seizures
    - o Sudden Death (?? Cardiac related)
    - o Neuroleptic Malignant Syndrome – NMS (very rare, but untreated has a high mortality)

25

- **TYPICAL ANTIPSYCHOTICS (1ST GENERATION ANTIPSYCHOTICS)**
  - **Chlorpromazine (Thorazine®)[154]**
    - 92-97% protein binding
    - Rare cholestatic jaundice (0.5%)
    - Hyperglycemia, photosensitivity (3%)
    - IM injection can be painful
    - Useful for hiccups and n/v
  - **Thioridazine (Mellaril®)[155]**
    - Highest of all neuroleptics in anticholinergic side effects
    - Lowest of all neuroleptics in EPS
    - Black Box Warning about QTc prolongation
    - Max dose 800 mg/d due to pigmentary retinopathy
    - Up to 60% incidence of retrograde ejaculation and other sexual dysfunction

> **RELATIVE POTENCIES:**
> *(lowest to highest)*
> 100mg Chlorpromazine (Thorazine) =
> 100mg Thioridazine (Mellaril)
> 50mg Mesoridazine (Serentil)
> 10mg Molindone (Moban)
> 10mg Loxapine (Loxitane)
> 8-10mg Perphenazine (Trilafon)
> 5mg Trifluoperazine (Stelazine)
> 4-5mg Thiothixene (Navane)
> 2mg Haloperidol (Haldol)
> 2mg Fluphenazine (Prolixin)

  - **Mesoridazine (Serentil®)[156]**
    - Metabolite of thioridazine
    - Potent antiemetic
    - Black Box Warning about QTc prolongation
    - Low EPS, high sedative and anticholinergic effects
    - Avoid excessive sunlight (photosensitivity)
  - **Molindone (Moban®)[157]**
    - Moderate EPS, low sedation and anticholinergic effects
    - Only agent reported not to cause weight gain
    - Less effect on lowering seizure threshold
    - Contraindications: severe cardiovascular disorders
  - **Loxapine (Loxitane®)[158]**
    - Active metabolite is amoxapine (Ascendin®)
    - Moderate EPS/anticholinergic effects
    - Low weight gain
    - Inhaled loxapine powder (Adasuve®) was FDA approved 12/2012 only through a restricted program under a Risk Evaluation and Mitigation Strategy (REMS) called the ADASUVE REMS because of risk of bronchospasm (precaution in respiratory patients)
      - Made by Alexza Pharmaceuticals and indicated for the acute treatment of agitation associated with schizophrenia or bipolar I disorder in adults
      - Dose is 10mg (thermal aerosolizer), peaks in 2 minutes, similar to an injection
  - **Perphenazine (Trilafon®)[159]**
    - Mid-potency
    - Also used to treat intractable hiccups and n/v
  - **Trifluoperazine (Stelazine®)[160]**
    - Also has anxiolytic indication
    - Dosing is BID up to QID
  - **Thiothixene (Navane®)[161]**
    - High potency, high EPS, moderate anticholinergic effects
  - **Haloperidol (Haldol®)[162]**
    - Very little anticholinergic side effects, high EPS, less sedation, little CV effects
    - Available as a decanoate in sesame oil[163]
      - Administered Q 4 weeks dosing via Z-track injection method
      - Dosed at 10-20 times the total daily oral dose
      - Give no more than 100mg on first dose (Z-track method), then give the rest in 3-7 days
      - Maximum volume per injection site – 3ml
      - Maximum dose – 450mg / month
    - Protect oral dosage forms from light
  - **Fluphenazine (Prolixin®)[164]**
    - High EPS
    - Available as a decanoate/IM depot in sesame oil[165]
      - Injected Q 2-3 weeks at 1.25 times the total daily oral dose (max 100mg/dose)
      - Given via Z-track injection method or Subcutaneous administration possible
    - Contraindications: sub-cortical brain damage, comatose, or severely depressed states
    - Monitoring: routine CBC w/diff due to incidence of blood dyscrasias

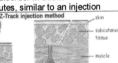

Z-Track injection method

Use side of hand to pull tissue to one side

- **ATYPICAL ANTIPSYCHOTICS – Work on multiple symptoms of schizophrenia**
  - **Clozapine (Clozaril®, Fazaclo® - orally disintegrating tablet)[166,167]**
    - Indicated for *Treatment-Resistant Schizophrenia* and to *reduce the risk of suicidal behavior* in schizophrenia/schizoaffective disorder
      - A pt must fail $\geq$ 3 antipsychotics over 5 yrs at adequate doses of >6 wks duration
      - To reduce suicide risk, patients must be continued for > 2 years of therapy
    - Structural analogue of Loxapine
    - D1 > D2, D4, 5HT2, 5HT3, 5HT6, and 5HT7 antagonist

- Also blocks alpha2, cholinergic, histaminic receptors
- Pregnancy Category B
- Dosing: 25-900 mg/d (slow titration)
- Very little EPS
- Side effects: drowsiness, dizziness, reflex tachycardia, orthostatic hypotension, N/V, fever, visual disturbances, constipation, weight gain, salivation, hyperglycemia, myocarditis (1%)
- Dose-related seizures (600-900mg: 5-14%) – especially from a rapid titration[168]
- RARE: agranulocytosis (0.38-0.73%) -- Requires weekly monitoring of WBCs for first six months, then Q 2 weeks for the next six months, then Q 4 weeks thereafter
- Clozapine blood levels > 350ng/ml preferred with clozapine:norclozapine ratio > 2:1[169,170,171,172,173,174]
- Cigarette smoking (P450-1A2 inducer) will ↑ metabolism, so larger doses may be needed

- **Risperidone (Risperdal®/ Risperdal® M Tabs/Risperdal Consta®)[175]**
  - D2 antagonist (affects positive symptoms) and 5HT2a antagonist (affects negative symptoms)
  - alpha1 and alpha2 blockade (see Remeron info)
  - Half-life is approx. 20 hours
  - Side effects: Sedation, orthostatic hypotension, dose-related EPS (No anticholinergic effects)
  - Available as 0.25mg, 0.5mg, 1mg, 2mg, 3mg, & 4mg tablets, liquid (1mg/ml) and Consta
  - Average dose is 4mg/d (National average)
  - Approved for Bipolar (ages 10-17) and Schizophrenia (ages 13-17) in adolescents
  - Risperdal® Consta® kit – Extended-release microspheres - IM Depot formulation[176]
    - Approved for Bipolar Disorder with or without Li+ / valproate
    - IM gluteal injection (12.5-25mg) (Max is 50mg) given every 2 weeks
    - Store in refrigerator (or out for up to 7 days), protected from light / needs reconstitution

- **Paliperidone (Invega®)[177]** – major metabolite of risperidone
  - Extended-release once daily dosing (OROS system)
    - Tablets should not be chewed or crushed; may see tablet shell in stool
  - Less EPS than risperidone
  - Approved for Schizophrenia (ages 12-17) in adolescents
  - Available as 3mg, 6mg, & 9mg extended release tablets
  - Recommended dose: 6mg/d -- Max dose: 12mg/d
  - Invega® Sustenna® (paliperidone palmitate) extended-release injectable suspension[178]
    - Initial dose of 234mg on day 1 and then 156mg one week later
      - Administered in the deltoid or gluteal muscle
    - Recommended monthly maintenance dose is 117mg (range 39-234mg)

- **Olanzapine (Zyprexa®/Zydis®)[179]**
  - Approved for acute Bipolar treatment and maintenance (incl. child/adolescents)
  - Structural analogue of clozapine
  - 93% protein bound
  - Dosing: 2.5-20 mg daily *(higher doses well tolerated)*
  - Side effects: drowsiness, dizziness, akathisia, weight gain
  - Cigarette smoking (P450-1A2 inducer) and valproic acid[180] will ↑ metabolism, so larger doses may be needed
  - Available in a rapidly acting IM injection
    - Must be reconstituted with 2.1ml of sterile water (makes 5mg/ml concentration)
    - Dose is 10mg which can be repeated in 2-4 hours – Max. of 3 injections (30mg)
    - Do not give within 1 hour of a Benzodiazepine – leads to bradycardia
  - Available in long-acting IM depot – Zyprexa Relprevv®[181]
    - BLACK BOX WARNING: Severe sedation (including coma) and/or delirium after each injection (0.1% incidence),so patient must be observed for at least 3 hours in a registered facility with ready access to emergency response services
    - Zyprexa Relprevv® is available only through a restricted distribution program
    - Doses: 150mg/2 wks, 300mg/4 wks, 210mg/2 wks, 405mg/4 wks, or 300mg/2 wks
    - Availability: Powder for suspension for IM use only: 210 mg/vial, 300 mg/vial, and 405 mg/vial

- **Quetiapine (Seroquel®)[86]**
  - Approved for Bipolar Depression, pediatric patients, and add-on for MDD
  - Structural analogue of clozapine
  - 83% protein bound
  - Partially metabolized by P450-3A4
  - Drug interactions: Phenytoin ↑s quetiapine clearance by 500%
  - Side effects: dizziness, postural hypotension, drowsiness, dry mouth, ↑ lipids, wt. gain
  - Little to no EPS or prolactin elevations seen across dose range
  - Dosing: Initiate at 50-100 mg BID; average: 600-800 mg/d *(higher doses well tolerated)*
  - Seroquel XR is dosed QD in the evening without food or with a light snack

- **Ziprasidone (Geodon®)[25]**
  - 5HT2a, 5HT2c, 5HT1d antagonist/5HT1a agonist > D2, D3 antagonist; moderate alpha1, histamine1 blockade and 5HT, NE reuptake inhibition
  - Up to two-fold absorption ↑ with food (Dose it at MEAL times)
  - Dosing: Initiate at 20 mg BID with food; average dose: 160 mg/d divided BID with food
  - > 99% protein bound
  - Side effects: ↑ QT interval, akathisia, anorexia, depression, diarrhea, hallucinations, headache, hostility, insomnia, N/V, rash
  - Drug interactions: drugs that prolong QT interval (quinidine, sotalol, thioridazine, etc.); carbamazepine ↓ levels 36%; ketoconazole ↑ levels 33%
  - Metabolized by P450-3A4; weak inhibitor of P450-2D6 (high dose)
  - EKG recommended in patients at high risk for cardiac complications

- **Aripiprazole (Abilify®)[182]**
  - Also approved for Adjunctive treatment of Depression / Bipolar
  - Partial dopamine agonist, 5HT1a agonist; 5HT2a antagonist; moderate alpha1, H1 blockade
  - > 99% protein bound
  - VERY LONG half-life: 75hrs + 96hrs for active metabolite
  - Metabolized by P450-2D6 and P450-3A4
  - Approved for bipolar (ages 10-17) and schizophrenia (ages 13-17) in adolescents
  - Side effects: headache, anxiety, insomnia, N/V, lightheadedness, akathisia, constipation
  - Dosing: 10-15 mg/d (up to 30mg/d) usually given in the AM due to insomnia/stimulation
  - Immediate-acting IM injection is 9.75 mg in 1.3 mL sterile water (max of 3 injections a day)

- **Iloperidone (Fanapt®)[26]**
  - Available in 1 mg, 2 mg, 4 mg, 6 mg, 8 mg, 10 mg and 12 mg tablets
  - Target dosage is 12 to 24mg per day divided BID (titrate slowly to reduce orthostatic hypotension)
  - Side effects: Dizziness, dry mouth, fatigue, nasal congestion, orthostatic hypotension, somnolence, tachycardia, and weight gain
  - Not a first-line agent due to QTc prolongation

- **Asenapine (Saphris®)[183]** – also approved for Bipolar
  - Available in 5mg and 10mg sublingual tablets (black cherry flavored)
    - For Schizophrenia: 5mg SL BID / For Bipolar Disorder: 10 mg SL BID
    - Administration: Food and water should be avoided for 10 minutes after dissolving the tablet under the tongue. Do not swallow the tablet.
  - Elimination of asenapine is primarily through direct glucuronidation by UGT1A4 and oxidative metabolism by cytochrome P450 isoenzymes (predominantly P450-1A2)
  - Caution if given with QTc-prolonging medications or in cardiac-risk patients
  - Serious allergic reactions have been reported to the FDA

- **Lurasidone (Latuda®)[184]**
  - Pregnancy Category B
  - Half-life is approximately 18 hrs
  - Metabolized via P450-3A4 to 2 active and 2 inactive metabolites
  - Dosage: 40mg to 160mg ONCE DAILY with FOOD (at least 350 calories)
    - Food increases absorption by 2-3 times
    - Available in 20mg, 40mg, 80mg and 120mg tablets
    - Dose should not exceed 40mg/d in those with severe hepatic/renal impairment (CrCl<50mL/min)
  - Common side effects: dose-related akathisia, nausea, somnolence, pseudoparkinsonism
  - Contraindicated with ketoconazole (can ↑ levels) and rifampin (can ↓ levels)
  - Caution with Diltiazem – Latuda dose should not exceed 40mg/d

---

- ★ **Combining Benzodiazepines + Antipsychotics work the fastest in decreasing psychotic aggression and acute manic symptoms**
  - For prn use only

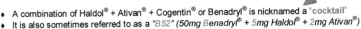

- A combination of Haldol® + Ativan® + Cogentin® or Benadryl® is nicknamed a "cocktail"
- It is also sometimes referred to as a "B52" (50mg Benadryl® + 5mg Haldol® + 2mg Ativan®)

USEFUL INFORMATION:[31,32,185,186,187]
- All Atypicals are effective for Bipolar disorder
- **Dementia** – Black Box Warning with atypical antipsychotics - ↑ **risk of death by 1.6-1.7X**
- All atypicals have the potential to cause weight gain and diabetes

RISK OF HYPERGLYCEMIA, WEIGHT GAIN, AND HYPERLIPIDEMIA
➔➔➔ ie. The Metabolic Syndrome
Risk of diabetes is 2-4x that of the non-psychiatric population (approx 13%)
Abilify, Geodon, Latuda < asenapine, Fanapt, Invega, Risperdal, Seroquel < Zyprexa, Clozaril
(almost alphabetical by Brand name)
➔Consensus guidelines from 2004 say that if patients develop diabetes or weight gain,
they should be switched to Geodon or Abilify[188]

RISK OF QTC PROLONGATION[189]
Mesoridazine > thioridazine > ziprasidone > iloperidone > haloperidol > quetiapine > clozapine >
risperidone > asenapine > olanzapine > paliperidone > aripiprazole > lurasidone

RISK OF PROLACTIN ELEVATIONS[190]
paliperidone > risperidone > *haloperidol (and other typicals)* > olanzapine >
quetiapine = ziprasidone = asenapine = lurasidone = iloperidone = aripiprazole = clozapine

DOSE-RELATED EPS
risperidone = paliperidone > olanzapine = ziprasidone = aripiprazole > quetiapine = clozapine

ORAL ANTIPSYCHOTICS:

Typical (1st Generation)	Atypical (2nd Generation)		
Low to High potency:		-apines:	-idones:
Chlorpromazine (Thorazine) Thioridazine (Mellaril) Mesoridazine (Serentil) Molindone (Moban) Loxapine (Loxitane) Perphenazine (Trilafon) Trifluoperazine (Stelazine) Thiothixene (Navane) Haloperidol (Haldol) Fluphenazine (Prolixin)	Aripiprazole (Abilify)	Loxapine (1st Gen) Clozapine (Clozaril) Olanzapine (Zyprexa) Quetiapine (Seroquel) Asenapine (Saphris)	Risperidone (Risperdal) Ziprasidone (Geodon) Paliperidone (Invega) Iloperidone (Fanapt) Lurasidone (Latuda)

INJECTABLE ANTIPSYCHOTICS:

Immediate-acting	
Typical:	**Atypical:**
Haldol Thorazine Numerous others	Geodon Abilify Zyprexa (no BZDs w/in 2 hrs)
Long-acting	
Typical:	**Atypical:**
Prolixin Decanoate (Q 2 weeks) Haldol Decanoate (Q 4 weeks)	Risperdal Consta (Q 2 weeks) Invega Sustenna (Q 4 weeks) Zyprexa Relprevv (Q 2-4 weeks)

ANTIPSYCHOTICS AND THEIR FDA-APPROVED INDICATIONS (AS OF 11/2012):

Indication: Antipsychotic:	Acute Bipolar	Bipolar Maintenance	Pediatric Bipolar	Pediatric Schizophrenia	Irritability in Autism	Adjunct in MDD
Abilify	✓ ±	✓	ages 10-17	ages 13-17	ages 6-17	✓
Fanapt						
Invega	S.A.D. ±			ages 12-17		
Invega Sustenna						
Latuda						
Risperdal	✓ ±		ages 10-17	ages 13-17	ages 5-16	
Risperdal Consta		✓ ±				
Saphris	✓ ±					
Seroquel	✓ ±	✓ ±	ages 10-17 ±	ages 13-17		
Seroquel XR	✓ ±	✓ +				✓
Zyprexa	✓ ±	✓	ages 13-17	ages 13-17		
Zyprexa Relprevv						

✓ = yes   ± = with or without adjunctive lithium or valproic acid
S.A.D. = Schizoaffective disorder   MDD = Major Depressive Disorder

LONG-ACTING INJECTABLES (LAI) CHART [163,165,176,178,181,191-193]

	Fluphenazine (Prolixin Decanoate®)	Haloperidol (Haldol Decanoate®)	Paliperidone Palmitate (Invega Sustenna®)	Risperidone (Risperdal Consta®)	Olanzapine (Zyprexa Relprevv®)
Dosing Options	25mg/ml sesame oil suspension for injection	50mg/ml & 100mg/ml sesame oil suspension for injection	Prefilled syringes containing: 39mg, 78mg, 117mg, 156, 234mg	Syringes that **require reconstitution** 12.5mg, 25mg, 37.5mg 50mg	210mg/vial 300mg/vial 405mg/vial
Indication	Schizophrenia	Schizophrenia	Schizophrenia	Schizophrenia Bipolar Type I (Mono or adjunctive therapy)	Schizophrenia
Admin-istration	IM injection q3 wks PO overlap: 0-7 days Initial dose: 1.2 x PO dose. Dose adjustments in increments of 12.5mg	IM injection q4 wks PO overlap: 1-3 wk Initial dose: 10-15 x PO; Not to Exceed 100mg for 1st dose.	IM injection q4 wks PO overlap: NONE Initial dose: 234mg x 1 dose (deltoid); 156mg once a week later; 117mg (maintenance dose) 3 weeks after 2nd dose.	IM injection q2 wks (max dose should not exceed 50mg q 2wks) PO overlap: 3 wks Initial dose: 2mg PO ≈ 25mg 4mg PO ≈ 50mg 6mg PO ≈ 75mg (Eerdekens et al, 2004)[194]	IM injection q2-4 wks PO overlap: NONE Initial dose: 150 to 210mg q2wks (10mg PO=150mg q2wks OR 300mg q4wks) (15mg PO=210mg q2 weeks OR 405mg q4wks (20mg PO = 300mg q2wks)
Onset of Action	≈ 24 to 72 hours	≈ 6 days	≈ a few hours	≈ 3 Weeks	≈ a few hours
Clinical Pearls	More painful injection; monitor for EPS	More painful injection; monitor for EPS	More difficult to dose due to 2 separate loading dose injections Renal dosing CI in renal pts of CrCl < 50ml/min	A 3 wk overlap of risperidone is clinically necessary	PDSS-Post Injection Delirium Sedation Syndrome risk (0.1%) will limit use (along with multiple registrations)

For patients who have never taken oral paliperidone or oral or injectable risperidone, tolerability should be established with oral paliperidone or oral risperidone prior to initiating treatment with INVEGA SUSTENNA[178].
- **Switching from Long-Acting Injectable Antipsychotics-**When switching patients from previous long-acting injectable antipsychotics, initiate INVEGA SUSTENNA therapy in place of the next scheduled injection. INVEGA SUSTENNA should then be continued at monthly intervals. The recommended initiation regimen (234 mg/156 mg paliperidone palmitate on Day 1/Day 8 as deltoid intramuscular injections) is not required.

APPROXIMATE DOSES NEEDED FOR SIMILAR ACTIVE MOIETY EXPOSURE[194]

RISPERDAL oral QD	RISPERDAL CONSTA IM Q2W	INVEGA SUSTENNA IM Q4W
1mg	12.5mg	39mg
2mg	25mg	78mg
4mg	37.5mg	117mg
5mg	50mg	156mg
6mg	75mg	195mg
>6mg	>75mg	234mg

SUBSTANCE-RELATED DISORDERS[195-197]

I. DEFINITIONS
   A. Drug Abuse – maladaptive or dangerous mis-use of a substance, without implying dependence
   B. Dependence – with abstinence, an individual experiences pathologic symptoms and signs
   C. Addiction – compulsive substance use & inability to control intake despite negative consequences
      – *Drug addiction is a disease!*

II. DRUGS OF ABUSE THAT CAN BE DETOXED
   A. Alcohol Withdrawal
      1. Phase I – Begins within hours and lasts 3-5 days
         – Autonomic hyperactivity (tachycardia, diaphoresis, labile blood pressure, anxiety, nausea and vomiting)
      2. Phase II – Perceptual disturbances, auditory or visual hallucinations
      3. Phase III – seizures (clonic-tonic) lasting 30 seconds to 4 minutes
      4. Phase IV – *delirium tremens*, occurs in < 1% of patients
   B. Benzodiazepines and other sedative-hypnotics
      1. Short-acting, lipophilic drugs are preferred agents of abuse
      2. Withdrawal times and severity depend on the half-life, amount, and time of abuse
   C. Opiates – Withdrawal times range from 3 to 14 days, depending on half-life of drug

III. DRUGS OF ABUSE THAT CANNOT BE DETOXED
   A. Angel Trumpet and other anticholinergics, PCP (Angel dust), Cocaine, Marijuana, Ecstasy, amphetamines, ketamine, LSD, mushrooms, steroids, Triple C's (nickname for Coricidin Cough & Cold – ie. Dextromethorphan), inhalants, Bath Salts, K2/Spice (synthetic marijuana)
   B. http://www.erowid.org/psychoactives/psychoactives.shtml

IV. WITHDRAWAL – Symptoms seen are usually the opposite of the abused drug

V. TREATMENT OF WITHDRAWAL
   A. Alcohol – can be life-threatening
      1. Give Vitamin B1 100mg (thiamine) to prevent Wernicke's encephalopathy
      2. Give multivitamin supplement and Folic Acid 1mg po QD
      4. Detox is done with a benzodiazepine to prevent seizures and DT's
         a. Chlordiazepoxide or diazepam are preferred (long-acting)
         b. LOT (lorazepam, oxazepam, temazepam) used in severe liver impairment
         c. Taper drug over 3-7 days
         d. Do not treat seizures with an anticonvulsant – use a benzo or similar
   B. Benzodiazepines – Detox and risks are similar to alcohol detox (use long-acting benzos)
   C. Opiates[198]
      1. Withdrawal is not life-threatening (unless severely medically compromised)
      2. Buprenorphine (Suboxone/Subutex) or Methadone taper by 5-10mg/d
      3. Clonidine – attenuates the noradrenergic hyperactivity of withdrawal
         a. Start at 0.1 to 0.2mg Q6h and taper over 5-7 days
         b. Watch for orthostatic hypotension and hypotension/bradycardia

VI. TREATMENT OF SUBSTANCE DEPENDENCE (AFTER DETOXIFICATION)
   A. Alcohol dependence
      1. Disulfiram (Antabuse®)[199] - Irreversibly inhibits aldehyde dehydrogenase
         a. Reaction can cause flushing, n/v, headache, palpitations, sweating, fever, MI, hypotension, respiratory depression, arrhythmias, CV collapse, and death
         b. Caution with any alcohol (cough syrups, mouthwashes)
         c. Dosed at 250mg to 500mg QD
      2. Naltrexone (Revia®)[200] – 50mg QD with food
         a. Blocks opiate receptors that are stimulated by endogenous opiates released while drinking alcohol
         b. Also used for opiate addictions
         c. Monthly depot IM injections are available (Vivitrol®)[201]
            1. Dose is 380 mg delivered intramuscularly every 4 weeks or once a month
      3. Acamprosate (Campral®)[202] delayed-release tablets
         a. Synthetic analog of GABA and taurine
         b. Dosed at two – 333mg tablets po TID (2gm a day divided)
         c. Renally eliminated, so safe in liver failure patients
         d. Side effects: Headache, GI symptoms, palpitations, peripheral edema
   B. Opiate dependence
      1. Methadone
      2. Buprenorphine (Suboxone®, Subutex®)[203] / Buprenorphine pellet SubQ (Titan Pharmaceuticals submitted a New Drug Application (NDA) to the FDA in October 2012 for Probuphine®)

INTOXICATION / DETOXIFICATION INFORMATION

MINOR ALCOHOL WITHDRAWAL	MAJOR ALCOHOL WITHDRAWAL (DTs)
Anorexia	Extreme restlessness
Diaphoresis	Fever
Diarrhea	Gross tremors
Elevated blood pressure	Increased psychomotor activity
Generalized weakness	Profound disorientation
Insomnia	Profuse diaphoresis
Nausea and vomiting	Tachycardia
Perception disorder	Vivid hallucinations
-nightmares, illusions, hallucinations	
Seizures	
Tachycardia	
Tremors	

BENZODIAZEPINE AND ALCOHOL INTOXICATION

Ataxia	Impaired attention	
Confusion	Loquacity	
Diminished reflexes	Mood changes	**Mild intoxication can
Euphoria or irritability	Nystagmus	cause disinhibition
Flushed face	Somnolence	
Hypotension Coma	Slurred speech	

OPIATE INTOXICATION	OPIATE WITHDRAWAL
Apathy	Diaphoresis
Attention impairment	Diarrhea
Dysphoria	Fever
Euphoria	Insomnia
Miosis	Lacrimation
Motor retardation	Muscle aching
Sedation	Mydriasis
Slurred speech	Piloerection
	Rhinorrhea
COCAINE INTOXICATION	Yawning
Elation / Euphoria	
Elevated or lowered blood pressure	**COCAINE WITHDRAWAL**
Grandiosity	Depression
Hypervigilance	Fatigue
Loquacity	Increased appetite
Motor agitation	Nightmares
Mydriasis	Sleep disturbance
Nausea and Vomiting	
Sweating or chills	
Tachycardia	

HALLUCINOGEN INTOXICATION

PSYCHOLOGICAL	PHYSICAL
Perceptual intensification	Mydriasis
Depersonalization	Tachycardia
Derealization	Diaphoresis
Illusions	Palpitations
Hallucinations	Blurred vision
Synesthesias	Tremor
Incoordination	
Dizziness	
Weakness	
Drowsiness	
Paresthesias	

MARIJUANA INTOXICATION

Apathy	Hallucinations
Conjunctival congestion	Increased appetite
Dry mouth	Sensory Intensification
Euphoria	Tachycardia

NICOTINE WITHDRAWAL

Anxiety	Irritability
Difficulty concentrating	Restlessness
Headache	Sleep disturbances
Increased appetite	

ANTICHOLINERGIC INTOXICATION

Ataxia	Mydriasis
Constipation	Tachycardia
Dry mouth	Warm dry skin

EFFECTS AT SPECIFIC BLOOD ALCOHOL CONCENTRATIONS

Alcohol can have different effects on different individuals, depending on their tolerance and biological sensitivity to alcohol. An individual's body size may not be a factor in their susceptibility to becoming easily intoxicated. Below, a Blood Alcohol Concentration (BAC) can be converted from % to actual concentration by multiplying by 1000.

0.02-0.03 BAC: (20-30mg/dl) Mild loss of coordination, slight euphoria and loss of shyness. Depressant effects are not apparent. Mildly relaxed and maybe a little lightheaded.

0.04-0.06 BAC: (40-60mg/dl) Feeling of well-being, relaxation, lower inhibitions, sensation of warmth. Euphoria. Some minor impairment of reasoning and memory, lowering of caution. Behaviors may become exaggerated and emotions intensified (Good emotions are better, bad emotions are worse)

0.07-0.09 BAC: (70-90mg/dl) Slight impairment of balance, speech, vision, reaction time, and hearing. Euphoria. Judgment and self-control are reduced, and caution, reason and memory are impaired, 0.08% is legally impaired and it is illegal to drive at this level. The person believes they are functioning better than they really are.

0.10-0.125 BAC: (100-125mg/dl) Significant impairment of motor coordination and loss of good judgment. Speech may be slurred; balance, vision, reaction time and hearing will be impaired. Euphoria.

0.13-0.15 BAC: (130-150mg/dl) Gross motor impairment and lack of physical control. Blurred vision and major loss of balance. Euphoria is reduced and dysphoria (anxiety, restlessness) is beginning to appear. Judgment and perception are severely impaired.

0.16-0.19 BAC: (160-190mg/dl) Dysphoria predominates and nausea may appear. The drinker has the appearance of a "sloppy drunk."

0.20 BAC: (200mg/dl) Felling dazed, confused or otherwise disoriented. Person may need help to stand or walk. Drinker may injure self and may not feel the pain. Some people experience nausea and vomiting at this level. The gag reflex is impaired and drinker can choke if vomiting. Blackouts are likely at this level (may not remember what has happened).

0.25 BAC: (250mg/dl) All mental, physical and sensory functions are severely impaired. Increased risk of asphyxiation from choking on vomit and of seriously injuring self by falls or other accidents.

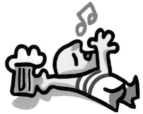

0.30 BAC: (300mg/dl) STUPOR. Drinker has little comprehension of where they are. Drinker may pass out suddenly and be difficult to awaken.

0.35 BAC: (350mg/dl) Coma is possible. This is the level of surgical anesthesia.

0.40 BAC and up: (>400mg/dl) Onset of coma, and possible death due to respiratory arrest.

URINE DETECTION OF DRUGS[204,205]

AGENT	TIME DETECTABLE IN URINE	DRUGS THAT CAN CAUSE FALSE POSITIVES
Alcohol	12 to 24 hours	Short-chain alcohols (eg. isopropyl alcohol)
Amobarbital	2 to 4 days	Ibuprofen, naproxen
Amphetamine	2 to 4 days	Trazodone, chlorpromazine, promethazine, pseudoephedrine, ranitidine, amantadine, bupropion, l-deprenyl, ephedrine, labetalol, selegiline, desipramine, phenylpropanolamine
Butalbital	2 to 4 days	Ibuprofen, naproxen
Cocaine (benzoylecgonine)	12 to 72 hours	
Codeine	2 to 4 days	Some quinolone antibiotics
Chlordiazepoxide	30 days	Sertraline, oxaprozin
Diazepam	30 days	Sertraline, oxaprozin
Dilaudid	2 to 4 days	
Heroin (morphine)	2 to 4 days	Poppy seeds, dextromethorphan, rifampin
Hydrocodone/Oxycodone	2 to 4 days	Some quinolone antibiotics
Hydromorphone	2 to 4 days	
Marijuana (Cannabinoids)		Ibuprofen, naproxen, dronabinol, efavirenz, proton pump inhibitors, tolmetin
-Occasional use	2 to 7 days	
-Regular use	30 days	
Methamphetamine	2 to 4 days	Brompheniramine, phenylpropanolamine, bupropion
Methadone	30 days	Diphenhydramine, doxylamine, quetiapine, chlorpromazine, verapamil
Morphine	2 to 4 days	
Pentobarbital	2 to 4 days	Ibuprofen, naproxen
Phencyclidine (PCP)		Venlafaxine, high dose ibuprofen, dextromethorphan, doxylamine, imipramine, ketamine, meperidine, tramadol, mesoridazine, thioridazine
-Occasional use	2 to 7 days	
-Regular use	30 days	
Phenobarbital	30 days	Ibuprofen, naproxen
Secobarbital	2 to 4 days	Ibuprofen, naproxen
Tricyclic Antidepressants	2 to 7 days	Carbamazepine, cyclobenzaprine, cyproheptadine, diphenhydramine, hydroxyzine, quetiapine

The periods of detection for the various abused drugs listed above should be taken as estimates since the actual figures will vary due to metabolism, user, laboratory, and excretion. All drug screens have a minimally detectable threshold established. If the concentration is below that threshold, the result is negative. If above, then positive. Thresholds may be determined by law.

COMMON METABOLIC PATHWAYS FOR OPIATES:

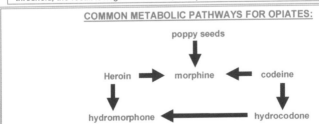

1) A False Negative Drug Screen happens when the drug is present but the levels are below the threshold of detection or are not part of the screening panel.
2) A Urine Drug Screen does not detect synthetic opioids (Fentanyl, Demerol, Ultram).
3) Oxycodone and Methadone are synthetic opiates but are included as separate tests in UDAS panel.

OPIOID COMPARISON CHART (EQUIANALGESIC DOSING)[206,207]

DRUG	☆	PEAK (hours)	EQUIVALENT DOSE (mg) SC / IV | PO		HALF-LIFE	DURATION OF ACTION	COMMENTS
AGONISTS							
Codeine	N	1 PO / 0.25-0.5 IM	100-130	200	2-3	2-6	Portion is demethylated to morphine / May be combined with non-opioid
Fentanyl (Duragesic®, Sublimaze®, Actiq®)	S	0.5 IM	0.05-0.2	-	1-2	1-6 SL / patch 72	Chest wall rigidity
Hydromorphone (Dilaudid®)	SS	1.5-2 PO / 0.5-1 IM	1.5-2	7.5	2-4	2-5	No active metabolite / Can be given rectally
Levorphanol (Levo-Dromoran®)	SS	1.5-2 PO / 0.5-1 IM	1-2	4	12-16	4-8	
Meperidine (Demerol®)	S	1-2 PO / 0.5-1 IM	75-100	300	2-5	2-4	Nor-meperidine toxicity limits utility
Methadone (Dolophine®)	S	1.5-2 PO / 0.5-1 IM	7.5-10	15-20	15-25	3-8	Accumulation = longer t½
Morphine	N	1.5-2 PO / 0.5-1 IM	10	60	2-3.5	3-7 / CR 8-12	Histamine release
Oxycodone (Percocet®, Percodan®, Oxycontin®, others)	SS	0.5-1 PO	-	15-20	2-3	2-6	May be combined with non-opioid
Oxymorphone (Numorphan®)	SS	1.5-2 PO / 0.5-1 IM	1-1.5	10-15	2-3	3-6	Can be given rectally
Hydrocodone (Vicodin® / Lortab®, others)	SS	0.5-1 PO	-	30	3.8	4-6	
Heroin (diacetylmorphine)	SS		5	60	2-4	2-4	
MIXED AGONIST-ANTAGONISTS		-- All are agonists at κ and σ receptors and antagonists at μ receptors					
Pentazocine (Talwin®)	S	1.5-2 PO / 0.5-1 IM	60	180	2-3	3-4	
Nalbuphine (Nubain®)	SS	0.5-1 IM	10-20	50-60	5	3-6	All can precipitate withdrawal in patients addicted to opioid agonists
Butorphanol (Stadol®)	S	0.5-1 IM	2	-	2.5-3.5	3-4	
PARTIAL AGONIST							
Buprenorphine (Suboxone®, Buprenex®, Butrans®, Subutex®)	SS	2-3 SL / 0.5-1 IM	0.3-0.6	0.4-0.8 SL	2-3	6-9	Can precipitate withdrawal in patients addicted to opioid agonists

☆→ N = Natural / S = Synthetic / SS = Semi-Synthetic

35

SPECIAL POPULATIONS AND ISSUES IN PSYCHIATRY

I. **PREGNANCY AND LACTATION**[70,71,74,75,208-217]
  → Benefits of medication must outweigh risks!!!
  - Mental illness poses a great risk to an unborn child and mother such as suicide, accidents, substance abuse, medical disorders, antepartum hemorrhaging, prematurity, low birth weight, and intrauterine growth retardation in the fetus
  - www.motherisk.org
  - Centre for Addiction and Mental Health handbook available at: http://www.camhx.ca/Publications/Resources_for_Professionals/Pregnancy_Lactation/psychmed_preg_lact.pdf
  ◆ Antidepressants:
    - Most are Category C, but Maprotiline is Category B
    - Paxil is Category D due to risk of CV malformations (Right ventricular obstructions)
    - SSRIs have small risk of Persistent Pulmonary Hypertension in the Newborn (PPHN)
      ▪ FDA reports that the SSRI link to PPHN is unclear because 2 studies say yes, but 3 say no
      ▪ SSRIs ↑ risk of pre-term birth and ↓ fetal head growth more than untreated depression[218,219]
    - 5-9% of mother's dose of Prozac is excreted in breast milk
      ▪ Most antidepressants can be used in breastfeeding with little problems if mother's need outweighs risk to infant
  ◆ Anxiolytics / BZDs ("like EtOH in a pill") – Category D and X
    - Small risk of cleft palate (controversial)
  ◆ Antipsychotics - All considered *relatively* safe in pregnancy
    - Watch for EPS or withdrawal in newborns (abnormal muscle movements)
    - Mostly Category C
    - Clozaril and Latuda are Category B
  ◆ Mood Stabilizers (Lithium, Depakote, Tegretol, Lamictal)
    - Mostly Category D (known teratogenic effects) especially if used in 1st trimester
      ▪ Folic Acid supplementation reduces the risk of neural tube malformations
    - Lithium – Ebstein's anomaly (displacement of the tricuspid valve)
    - Depakote – craniofacial defects, spina bifida (5-10X general population), cardiovascular & other malformations
      ▪ Children may have a 10 point lower IQ and an increased risk of having autism[80,81]
    - Tegretol – craniofacial defects, spina bifida, cardiovascular & other malformations
    - Lamictal is Category C but reports to FDA of up to 25X higher risk of cleft palate and other malformations have been seen – still the safest option for seizures
    - Can use atypical antipsychotics
    - 0-30% of mother's lithium dose is excreted in breast milk, so caution advised[220]

II. **CHILDREN AND ADOLESCENTS**[221-227]
  ◆ Antidepressants:
    - Prozac (ages 8-17) and Lexapro (ages 12-17) are the only FDA-approved newer agents
      ▪ Evidence-based support is lacking with other antidepressants for depression
    - Doxepin (ages ≥12) is FDA-approved, but TCAs have high cardiac risks
    - Imipramine (ages ≥6) is FDA-approved for bedwetting
    - Paxil should be avoided—suicidal ideation & "emotional lability" (2x as likely); short t1/2
      ▪ FDA has issued a warning against its use in children & adolescents
    - Effexor should be avoided—short t1/2
  ◆ OCD: Luvox (ages ≥8), Anafranil (ages ≥10), and Zoloft (ages ≥6) are FDA-approved
    ▪ Usually in OCD, highest possible doses are used to treat symptoms
  ◆ There is a similarity between ADHD and Bipolar disorder (symptoms appear alike)
    - Bipolar → have very long temper tantrums and graphically violent nightmares
  ◆ Anxiolytics: BZDs more likely to cause disinhibition and more abuse potential
  ◆ Antipsychotics:
    - Many atypicals approved in pediatric Bipolar and/or Schizophrenia (see pg. 29)
      ▪ Risperdal (ages 5-16) and Abilify (ages >6) FDA-approved for irritability in Autism
      ▪ Risperdal – increases Prolactin and ↑ risk of EPS
    - Haldol (ages ≥3), Mellaril (ages ≥2), and Orap (pimozide) (ages ≥12 for Tourette's)
  ◆ Mood Stabilizers:
    - Li+ approved – Not recommended for children under 12 yrs old (approved for ages ≥12)
      ▪ Must monitor for side effects and hypothyroidism
    - Depakote – monitor LFTs, platelets, polycystic ovarian syndrome (PCOS)
      ▪ Approved for ages >2 for seizures
    - Lamictal – ↑ incidence of rash; can progress to Stevens-Johnson; <u>MUST titrate slowly</u>!!!
      ▪ Beware of interactions affecting Lamictal with birth control pills
    - Carbamazepine – Drug interactions with oral contraceptives, hyponatremia, rash!!!
      ▪ Approved for any age for seizures

III. CONTRACEPTION AND PSYCHOTROPICS[209,212]

- ♦ Two methods of contraception are advised: hormonal and mechanical
- ♦ Combined oral contraceptives with high dose progestin if taking an enzyme-inducing drug
- ♦ Patients should take their pill continuously ("long cycle therapy")
- ♦ Avoid progestin-only pills and subdermal progestogen implants because likely to be ineffective if used with an enzyme inducing anti-epileptic drug (EI-AED)[228]
- ♦ Depot medroxyprogesterone acetate (MPA) should be effective, but may have serious side effects, such as delayed return to fertility and impaired bone health
- ♦ Levonorgestrel intrauterine system is effective, even with enzyme-inducing drugs
- ♦ IUDs and condoms avoid drug-drug interactions

IV. GERIATRIC PATIENTS

- ♦ UTIs, respiratory infections, and dehydration: can induce psychosis/delirium
- ♦ Dementia (typical and atypical antipsychotic black box warning) – 1.6-1.7x ↑ risk of death (CV, infection)[185,187]
  - Atypicals still preferred over typical antipsychotics
  - Anticholinergic drugs can negate the benefits of cholinesterase inhibitors
  - Large study of > 5000 patients found 37% received 1 anticholinergic & 11% received ≥ 2[229]
- ♦ BEERS List/Criteria[230,231] - see www.fmda.org/beers.pdf
  - Benzodiazepines ↑ risk of hip fractures, dementia, disinhibition, and ↑ risk of death[232]

V. BIPOLAR DEPRESSION[59,60,61,64]

- ♦ "Mood stabilizers" vs. antidepressants vs. Symbyax (olanzapine + fluoxetine) vs. Seroquel
- ♦ Antidepressants should not be used alone; can induce mania and ↑ rate of cycling
- ♦ Wellbutrin has least likelihood of inducing mania (no 5HT effects)
- ♦ Seroquel approved for both mania and bipolar depression (can be used as monotherapy)

VI. SUBSTANCE ABUSE AND MENTAL HEALTH ISSUES[191,233,234,235]

- ♦ Hi co-occurrence between mental health and substance abuse
- ♦ Drugs preferred by users ("self-medication")
  - Anxiety & Depression (EtOH, marijuana, nicotine, BZDs)
    - EtOH – creates more depression
    - Nicotine – anxiolytic and stimulatory effects
  - Bipolar disorder (up to 60% abuse EtOH, marijuana, and/or cocaine)
  - Schizophrenia (cocaine, nicotine)
    - Cocaine – helps with ↑ attention, but the ↑ DA which can ↑ psychosis
    - Nicotine – 70-80% of schizophrenic patients smoke
  - Potency of substances will ↑ psychoactive effects and ↑ risk of abuse

VII. SUICIDE RISKS[225,226,227]

- ♦ Benefit of medication must outweigh risk
- ♦ Teenagers – have an ↑ risk of suicide / 2nd leading cause of death (15-24 y.o.'s)
- ♦ Suicide risks by disease state:
  - Bipolar disorder – 15%; (25-50% attempt); usually in depression phase or in transition
  - Schizophrenia – 20% (70% attempt)
  - Depression – 15-20%
- ♦ All antidepressants carry a Black Box warning of the risk of suicide when starting therapy

VIII. POLYPHARMACY

- ♦ Antipsychotics – use of multiple drugs is not justified in the medical literature[30,186,236,237]
  - Polypharmacy does not increase efficacy, only increases side effects
  - Quetiapine should not be used as a sleeping pill[238]
  - One meta-analysis found it may be superior under certain clinical situations[239]
    1. Polypharmacy must start before any treatment failures can be determined
    2. Use for > 10 weeks
    3. Use of a Typical and Atypical antipsychotic
    4. Can use Clozaril
    5. Used only in China on Chinese population
- ♦ Antidepressants – may be used if pt. has partial response once single agent maximized
  - Use agents from different classes
  - New evidence is building to support initial polypharmacy to achieve higher remission rates[240]
    - Remission rate with mirtazapine + fluoxetine or venlafaxine or bupropion was superior to fluoxetine alone (52% vs. 58% vs. 46% vs. 25% respectively)
    - Other studies show similar results using a TCA + SSRI, antidepressant + L-methylfolate, and antidepressant + benzodiazepine receptor agonist, although some disagree[241,242]
- ♦ Mood stabilizers – Studies show better results than single agent therapy
  - Li+, VPA, CBZ, Lamictal with an atypical antipsychotic
- ♦ Anxiolytics – Can use BZDs prn (short-term) with antidepressants until they start to work

IX. TREATMENT-RESISTANT DEPRESSION (TRD)[98,99]

- Occurs when a patient does not respond to an adequate course of 2 antidepressants
  - At least 6-12 weeks on each antidepressant at the maximally tolerated dose
- Combinations of antidepressants with differing mechanisms should be tried first
- FDA-approved therapies:
  - Symbyax (olanzapine + fluoxetine) – approved on 3/19/09
  - Abilify
  - Seroquel
  - Vagal nerve stimulation
  - Deplin® (L-methylfolate) – a "medical food"
- Standard Augmentation Techniques:
  - Lithium
  - Cytomel® 25-50 µg/day
  - Carbamazepine (Tegretol®)
  - Buspirone (BuSpar®)
  - Monoamine Oxidase Inhibitor + other Antidepressant [Caution!]
  - Electroconvulsive Therapy (ECT) - (6 to 12 exposures)

X. MEDICATION NON-ADHERENCE

- Estimated at > 50% in 1 year[243]
- Similar or higher than those with other chronic conditions requiring medication (ie. HTN/DM)
- Dosing frequency <u>directly</u> correlates to non-adherence
- Other factors of non-adherence
  - Polypharmacy
  - Cost of medication / insurance co-pays
  - Side effects
  - Disbelief in being mentally ill

XI. MEDICAL COMORBIDITIES AND MENTAL ILLNESS[244]

- Bipolar & Schizophrenia patients are 2x more likely to have diabetes than general population
  - Including increased risk of The Metabolic Syndrome: dyslipidemia, HTN, obesity
- Pts >65 y.o. have a 19% greater 1yr risk for mortality with any mental disorder after an MI
- Pts >65 y.o. have a 34% increased risk for mortality if they have schizophrenia[245]
- Some antipsychotics can increase risk of The Metabolic Syndrome, so monitoring of waist circumference, BMI, lipids, fasting glucose, HgA1C should be done periodically
- Smoking cessation counseling can reduce mortality risks at any age

POSSIBLE PHARMACOTHERAPEUTIC INTERVENTIONS

1. Polypharmacy:
   - Antidepressants (other than the addition of trazodone for sleep)
   - Antipsychotics (including Depots that are not the same as patient's p.o. antipsychotic)
2. Drug worsens side effects, which is then treated with another agent
3. Drug worsens one disease state when used to treat another
4. Dosing time of day (ie. Abilify should be dosed in AM because it is stimulating)
5. Dosing frequency (TID or BID when a drug should be given QD)
6. Drug used in child, which is not approved, over one that is approved
7. Off-label use of drug that has <u>no</u> evidence-based efficacy (ie. Some anticonvulsants in Bipolar Disorder)
8. Dose of Seroquel too low (ie. 25-100mg at HS for sleep)
9. Geodon given in kids or elderly (should have an EKG first)
10. Depakote proper monitoring (Platelets, LFTs, blood levels)
11. Lithium proper monitoring (WBCs, SrCr, electrolytes, blood levels)
12. Dementia patients – Are they receiving BZDs or anticholinergics?
13. Other Key Drug Levels:

Lithium – acute	→	0.8 – 1.2 mEq/L	→ Levels in 5 days
Lithium – maintenance	→	0.4 – 1.0 mEq/L	→ Levels in 5 days
Valproic acid	→	50 – 125 mcg/ml	→ Levels in 3 days
Carbamazepine	→	4 – 12 mcg/ml	→ Levels in 5 days, then recheck in 5 weeks due to auto-induction
Phenytoin	→	10 – 20 mcg/ml	→ Levels in 5 days
Phenobarbital	→	15 – 40 mcg/ml	→ Levels in 5 days
Nortriptyline	→	50 – 150 ng/ml	→ Levels in 5 days
Desipramine	→	125 – 300 ng/ml	→ Levels in 5 days

References

1. American Psychiatric Association. Diagnostic and Statistical Manual of Mental Disorders, 4th ed. Text revised (DSM-IV-TR). Washington DC. American Psychiatric Association. 2000.
2. King V, Robinson S, Bianco T, et al. Choosing antidepressants for adults: clinicians guide. Agency for Healthcare Research and Quality Advancing Excellence in Health Care. AHRQ Publication No. 07-EHC007-3. August 2007. http://www.effectivehealthcare.ahrq.gov
3. Solomon DA, Keller MB, Leon AC, et al. Multiple Recurrences of Major Depressive Disorder. The American Journal of Psychiatry Feb 2000;157(2):229-233.
4. Weilburg JB, O'Leary KM, Meigs JB, et al.: Evaluation of the adequacy of outpatient antidepressant treatment. Psychiatr Serv. 2003;54:1233-1239.
5. Ruhe HG MD, Huyser J MD, Swinkels JA, et al. Dose escalation for insufficient response to standard-dose selective serotonin reuptake inhibitors in major depressive disorder: Systematic review. British Journal of Psychiatry 189(4):309-316, October 2006.
6. Watanabe N, Omori IM, Nakagawa A, et al. Mirtazapine versus other antidepressants in the acute-phase treatment of adults with major depression: systematic review and meta-analysis. Journal of Clinical Psychiatry 69(9):1404-15, 2008 Sep.
7. Miyamoto S, Duncan G, Marx C, et al. Treatments for schizophrenia: a critical review of pharmacology and mechanisms of action of antipsychotic drugs. Molecular Psychiatry. 10(1):79-104, January 2005.
8. Webber M, Marder S. Better pharmacotherapy for schizophrenia: What does the future hold? Current Psychiatry Reports. 10(4):352-8, August 2008.
9. Gardner D, Baldessarini R, Waraich P. Modern antipsychotic drugs: a critical overview. CMAJ Canadian Medical Association Journal. 172(13):1703-1711, June 21, 2005.
10. Katzman M. Current Considerations in the Treatment of Generalized Anxiety Disorder. CNS Drugs. 23(2):103-120, January 2009.
11. Sramek J, Zarotsky V, Cutler Neal. Generalized Anxiety Disorder: Treatment Options. Drugs. 62(11):1635-1648, January 2002.
12. BuSpar®, buspirone [package insert]. Bristol-Myers Squibb Company, Princeton, NJ, 1998.
13. Thase ME. Maintenance therapy for bipolar disorder. Journal of Clinical Psychiatry. 69(11):e32, 2008 Nov.
14. Smith LA, Cornelius V, Warnock A, et al. Effectiveness of mood stabilizers and antipsychotics in the maintenance phase of bipolar disorder: a systematic review of randomized controlled trials. Bipolar Disorders. 9(4):394-412, June 2007.
15. Gelenberg AJ MD, Pies R MD. Matching the Bipolar Patient and Mood Stabilizer. Annals of Clinical Psychiatry. 15(3-4):203-216, September/December 2003.
16. Berk M and Malhi GS. Should antipsychotics take pole position in mania treatment? The Lancet October 8, 2011;378:1279-81.
17. Eskalith® Lithium [package insert]. GlaxoSmithKline, Research Triangle Park, NC, 2003.
18. Depakote®, Depakene® valproic Acid [package insert]. Abbott Laboratories, North Chicago, IL, 2006.
19. Tegretol®, Epitol®, Equetro™ carbamazepine [package insert]. Novartis Pharmaceuticals, East Hanover, NJ, 2007.
20. Dilantin® Kapseals® [package insert]. Parke-Davis, New York, NY, 2003.
21. Luminal® phenobarbital [package insert]. Eli Lilly and Company, Indianapolis, IN, 1995.
22. Nortriptyline [package insert]. Corona CA: Watson Laboratories, Inc.; 2007 August.
23. Desipramine [package insert]. Bridgewater, NJ: Sanofi-Aventis; 2007 July.
24. Zyvox® linezolid [package insert]. Pfizer, Pharmacia & Upjohn Co. New York, NY, 2012.
25. Geodon® ziprasidone [package insert]. Pfizer Inc, NY, NY, 2008.
26. Fanapt® iloperidone [package insert]. Novartis, East Hanover, NJ, 2012.
27. Wagner KD, Kowatch RA, Emslie GJ, et al. A double-blind, randomized, placebo-controlled trial of oxcarbazepine in the treatment of bipolar disorder in children and adolescents. Am J Psychiatry. 2006;163(7):1179-1186.
28. MacMillan CM, Korndorfer SR, Rao S, et al. A comparison of divalproex and oxcarbazepine in aggressive youth with bipolar disorder. Journal of Psychiatric Practice. 2006 Jul;12(4):214-222.
29. Correll CU, Frederickson AM, Kane JM, et al. Does antipsychotic polypharmacy increase the risk for metabolic syndrome? Schizophrenia Research 2007:89:91-100.
30. Ack Tranulis C, Skalli L, Lalonde P, et al. Benefits and Risks of Antipsychotic Polypharmacy: An Evidence-Based Review of the Literature. Drug Safety. 31(1):7-20, January 2008.
31. Girgis R, Javitch J, Lieberman J, et al. Antipsychotic drug mechanisms: links between therapeutic effects, metabolic side effects and the insulin signaling Pathway. Molecular Psychiatry. 13(10):918-929, October 2008.
32. Nasrallah, H. Atypical antipsychotic-induced metabolic side effects: insights from receptor-binding profiles. Molecular Psychiatry. 13(1):27-35, January 2008.
33. Ito H, Koyoma A, Higuchi T. Polypharmacy and excessive dosing: psychiatrists' perceptions of antipsychotic drug prescription. British Journal of Psychiatry. 187(3):243-247, September 2005.
34. Tune L, Carr S, Hoag E, et al. Anticholinergic effects of drugs commonly prescribed for the elderly. Am J Psych 1992; 149:1393-1394.
35. Sidney H. Kennedy, Henning F. Andersen, and Raymond W. Lam. Efficacy of escitalopram in the treatment of major depressive disorder compared with conventional selective serotonin reuptake inhibitors and venlafaxine XR: a meta-analysis. J Psychiatry Neurosci. 2006 March; 31(2): 122–131.
36. S. Svensson and P. R. Mansfield. Escitalopram: superior to citalopram or a chiral chimera? Psychother Psychosom. 2004 Jan-Feb;73(1):10-6.
37. S. K. Teo et al. Clinical pharmacokinetics of thalidomide. Clin Pharmacokinet. 2004;43(5):311-27.
38. Bystritsky A. Treatment-resistant anxiety disorders. Molecular Psychiatry. 11(9):805-814, September 2006.
39. Velotis C, Wodarski S. Highlights From Current Research on Anxiety Disorders: The Most Common Psychiatric Illnesses Affecting Children and Adults. PsycCRITIQUES. 50(42), October 2005.
40. Jongsma A, Nichols K. Comprehensive Treatment of Anxiety Disorders. PsycCRITIQUES. 49(Sup11), Dec. 2004.
41. Spett M. Treating Anxiety Disorders: Drugs, Psychotherapy, or Both? PsycCRITIQUES. 49 (Supplement 4), October 2004.

42. The National Institute of Mental Health (NIMH) website on Attention Deficit Hyperactivity Disorder (ADHD). Accessed on 2/6/2012 at http://www.nimh.nih.gov/health/topics/attention-deficit-hyperactivity-disorder-adhd/index.shtml
43. Jefferson B Prince , Peter S. Jensen, Amy Vierhile. Piecing together the ADHD Puzzle: Treatment Strategies for attention deficit Hyperactivity Disorder (ADHD) From Childhood to Adolescence and through the Transition years. Found at http://cme.medscape.com/viewprogram/6043. Accessed on 3/23/09.
44. Stephen V. Faraone, Norra MacReady, Highlights of the 2008 U.S. Psychiatric and Mental Health Congress. New Research on Pharmacologic Therapy in ADHD. Found at http://cme.medscape.com/viewprogram/17840_pnt. Accessed on 3/1/09.
45. Scott H. Kollins, Laurie E. Scudder, Elizabeth Samander. ADHD in Childhood and Adolescence: New Evidence in Diagnosis and Treatment. Found at http://cme.medscape.com/viewprogram/18705_pnt. Accessed on 3/23/09.
46. Habel LA, Cooper WO, Sox CM, et al. ADHD medications and risk of serious cardiovascular events in young and middle-aged adults. JAMA 2011 Dec 28;306(24):2673-83.
47. Cooper WO, Habel LA, Sox CM, et al. ADHD drugs and serious cardiovascular events in children and young adults. N Engl J Med 2011; 365:1896-1904.
48. Vitiello B, Elliott GR, Swanson JM, et al. Blood Pressure and Heart Rate Over 10 Years in the Multimodal Treatment Study of Children with ADHD. Am J Psychiatry 2012;169:167-177.
49. Strattera™ atomoxetine [package insert]. Indianapolis, IN: Ely Lily & Co.; 2005 November.
50. Wellbutrin® bupropion [package insert]. Research Triangle Park, NC: GlaxoSmithKline; 2007 August.
51. Catapres® clonidine [package insert]. Boehringer Ingelheim, Ridgefield, CT, 1998.
52. Kapvay® clonidine [package insert]. Shionogi Pharma, Inc., Atlanta, GA, 2010.
53. Intuniv™ guanfacine [package insert]. Shire US Inc., Wayne, PA, 2009.
54. Modafinil [package insert]. Frazer, PA: Cephalon, Inc.; 2005 November.
55. Medications used in the Treatment of ADHD. In: Managing Medication for Children and Adolescents with ADHD. National Resource Center on ADHD Children. A Program of CHADD. May 2011. http://www.help4adhd.org/documents/WWWK3.pdf
56. A.D.D Warehouse. Medication chart to treat attention deficit hyperactivity disorder. http://www.addwarehouse.com/shopsite_sc/store/html/article3.htm.
57. The official 2010 TCPR ADHD medication comparison chart. The Carlat Psychiatry Report October 2010. http://thecarlatreport.com/article/official-2010-tpcr-adhd-medication-comparison-chart
58. Gold Standard, Inc. Amphetamines (class) Clinical Pharmacology [database online]. Available at: http://www.clinicalpharmacology.com. Accessed: June 16, 2012.
59. Nierenberg AA. Effective agents in treating bipolar depression. J Clin Psy Oct 2008;69(10):e29.
60. Bond DJ, Noronha MM, Kauer-Sant'Anna, et al. Antidepressant-associated mood elevations in bipolar II disorder compared with bipolar I disorder and major depressive disorder a systematic review and meta-analysis. Journal of Clinical Psychiatry. 69(10):1589-601, 2008 Oct.
61. Goldberg JF, Ghaemi S, Nassir. Benefits and limitations of antidepressants and traditional mood stabilizers for treatment of bipolar depression. Bipolar Disorders Supplement. 7 (Supplement 5):3-12, December 2005.
62. Taylor MJ, Goodwin GM. Long-term prophylaxis in bipolar disorder. CNS Drugs. 2006;20(4):303-10.
63. Barnes C, Mitchell P. Considerations in the management of bipolar disorder in women. Aust N Z J Psychiatry. 2005 Aug;39(8):662-7.
64. Bourin M, Prica C. The role of mood stabilisers in the treatment of the depressive facet of bipolar disorders. Neurosci Biobehav Rev. 2007;31(6):963-75
65. Nolen WA. Anticonvulsants, Antidepressants and Traditional Mood Stabilisers: Review of the Latest Data. Bipolar Disorders. 10 (Supplement 1): 16, February 2008.
66. Davis JM, Janicak PG, Hogan DM. Mood stabilizers in the prevention of recurrent affective disorders: a meta-analysis. Acta Psychiatrica Scandinavia. 100(6):406-417, December 1999.
67. Kirov G, Tredget J, John R, Owen MJ, et al. A cross-sectional and a prospective study of thyroid disorders in lithium-treated patients. J Affect Disord. 2005 Aug;87(2-3):313-7.
68. McKnight RF, Adida M, Budge K, et al. Lithium toxicity profile: a systematic review and meta-analysis. The Lancet, Early Online Publication, 20 January 2012. doi:10.1016/S0140-6736(11)61516-X. Accessed on 1/20/2012 at www.thelancet.com.
69. Llewellyn A, Stowe ZN, Strader JR. The use of lithium and management of women with bipolar disorder during pregnancy and lactation. J Clin Psychiatry 1998;59 Suppl 6:57-64; discussion 65.
70. Ward S, Wisner KL. Collaborative management of women with bipolar disorder during pregnancy and postpartum: Pharmacological considerations. J Midwifery Womens Health 2007 Jan-Feb;52(1):3-13.
71. Iqbal MM, Sohhan T, Mahmud SZ. The effects of lithium, valproic acid, and carbamazepine during pregnancy and lactation. J Toxicol Clin Toxicol 2001;39(4):381-92.
72. Goodnick PJ, Chaudry T, Artadi J, Arcey S. Women's issues in mood disorders. Expert Opin Pharmacother 2000 Jul;1(5):903-16.
73. Sharma V. Management of bipolar II disorder during pregnancy and the postpartum period—Motherisk Update 2008. Can J Clin Pharmacology/Journal Canadian de Pharmacologic Clinique 2009;16(1):e33-41.
74. Gentile S. Prophylactic treatment of bipolar disorder in pregnancy and breastfeeding: focus on emerging mood stabilizers. Bipolar Disorders. 8(3):207-220, June 2006.
75. Mood stabilisers 'safe' to use while breastfeeding. Inpharma Weekly. (1232);5, April 8, 2000.
76. Terao T, Okuno K, Okuno T, et al. A simpler and more accurate equation to predict daily lithium dose. J Clin Psychopharmacol. 1999 Aug;19(4):336-40.
77. Zetin M, Garber G, De Antonio M et al. Prediction of lithium dose: a mathematical alternative to the test dose method. J Clin Psychiatry 1983;44:144-145.
78. Baldessarini RJ, Tondo L, and Hennen J. Treating the suicidal patient with bipolar disorder. Reducing suicide risk with lithium. Ann N Y Acad Sci. 2001 Apr;932:24-38; discussion 39-43.
79. Reed RC, Dutta S. Does it really matter when a blood sample for valproic acid concentration is taken following once-daily administration of divalproex-ER? Ther Drug Moni. 2006;28(3):413-8.
80. Meador KJ, Baker GA, Browning N, et al. Cognitive Function at 3 Years of Age after Fetal Exposure to Antiepileptic Drugs. N Engl J Med 2009; 360:1597-1605. April 16, 2009

81. Bromley RL, Mawer R, Clayton-Smith J, et al. Autism spectrum disorders following in utero exposure to antiepileptic drugs. Neurology December 2, 2008;71(23):1923-1924. doi: 10.1212/01.wnl.0000339399.64213.1a

82. Allen MH, Hirschfeld RM, Wozniak PJ, et al. Linear Relationship of Valproate Serum Concentration to Response and Optimal Serum Levels for Acute Mania. Am J Psychiatry 2006;163:272-275.

83. Lamictal®, Lamotrigine [package insert]. GlaxoSmithKline, Research Triangle Park, NC, 2007.

84. Harden CL, Herzog AG, Nikolov BG, et al. Hormone replacement therapy in women with epilepsy: a randomized, double-blind, placebo-controlled study. Epilepsia 2006;47(9):1447-1451.

85. Symbyax®, Olanzapine + Fluoxetine [package insert]. Eli Lilly and Company, Indianapolis, IN, 2009.

86. Seroquel® Quetiapine [package insert]. AstraZeneca Pharmaceuticals, Wilmington, DE, 2009.

87. Trileptal®, oxcarbazepine [package insert]. Novartis, East Hanover, NJ, 2007.

88. Wagner KD, Kowatch RA, Emslie GJ, et al. A double-blind, randomized, placebo-controlled trial of oxcarbazepine in the treatment of bipolar disorder in children and adolescents. Am J Psychiatry 2006 Jul;163(7):1179-86.

89. Perahia D, Pritchett YL, Kajdasz DK, et al. A randomized, double-blind comparison of duloxetine and venlafaxine in the treatment of patients with major depressive disorder. J Psych Research, 2007.

90. Pharmacist's Letter / Prescriber's Letter May 2008 ~ Volume 24 ~ Number 240509

91. Gartlehner G, Gaynes BN, Hansen RA, et al. Comparative benefits and harms of second-generation antidepressants: background paper for the American College of Physicians. Ann Intern Med. 2008 Nov 18;149(10):734-50.

92. Iqbal SH, Prashker M. Pharmacoeconomic Evaluation of Antidepressants: A Critical Appraisal of Methods. Pharmacoeconomics. 23(6):595-606, 2005.

93. Montgomery S, Doyle J, Stern L, et al. Economic Considerations in the Prescribing of Third-Generation Antidepressants. Pharmacoeconomics. 23(5):477-491, 2005.

94. Ereshefsky L, Jhee S, Grothe D. Antidepressant Drug-Drug Interaction Profile Update. Drugs in R&D. 6(6):323-336, 2005.

95. Norman TR, Olver JS. New Formulations of Existing Antidepressants: Advantages in the Management of Depression. CNS Drugs. 18(8):505-520, 2004.

96. Antidepressants: benefits overstated, harms understated? Inpharma Weekly. (1434):24, April 24, 2004.

97. Handbook of Psychiatric Drug Therapy, Sixth Edition, by Labbate LA, et al. (Lippincott Williams & Wilkins, Philadelphia, 2010, p. 54)

98. Thase ME. Effectiveness of Antidepressants: Comparative Remission Rates. Archives of General Psychiatry, 2005 Jun;62(6):617-27

99. Stahl SM. Why Settle for Silver, When You Can Go for Gold? Response vs. Recovery as the Goal of Antidepressant Therapy. Available at: http://www.psychiatrist.com/pcc/brainstorm/br6004.htm. Accessed on 10/18/2010.

100. Koga M, Kodaka F, Miyata H, and Nakayama K. Symptoms of delusion: the effects of discontinuation of low-dose venlafaxine. Acta Psychiatr Scand. 2009 October; 120(4): 329-331.

101. Warner CH, Bobo W, Warner C, Reid S, Rachal J. Antidepressant discontinuation syndrome. Am Fam Physician. 2006 Aug 1; 74(3):449-56.

102. Haddad P, Lejoyeux M, Young A. Title Antidepressant discontinuation reactions: Are preventable and simple to treat. BMJ. 1998 April; 316(7138):1105-1106.

103. Muzina DJ. Discontinuing an antidepressant? Tapering tips to ease distressing symptoms. Current Psychiatry. 2010 March; 9(3):51-61.

104. Fluoxetine [package insert]. Pomona, NY: Barr Laboratories, Inc.; 2008 March.

105. Sertraline [package insert]. Morgantown, WV: Mylan Pharmaceuticals, Inc.; 2008 Aug.

106. Paroxetine [package insert]. Sellersville, PA: Teva Pharmaceuticals; 2007 August.

107. Newport DJ, Stowe ZN. Clinical management of perinatal depression: focus on paroxetine. Psychopharmacol Bull. 2003 Spring;37 Suppl 1:148-66.

108. Fluvoxamine [package insert]. Sellersville, PA: Teva Pharmaceuticals; 2008 February.

109. Celexa® Citalopram [package insert]. Bonita Springs, FL: Forest Pharmaceuticals; 2011 August.

110. Lexapro® Escitalopram [package insert]. St. Louis, MO: Forrest Laboratories, Inc.; 2009 January.

111. Cymbalta® Duloxetine [package insert]. Indianapolis, IN: Eli Lilly & Co.; 2005 December.

112. Venlafaxine [package insert]. Sellersville, PA: Teva Pharmaceuticals; 2008 August.

113. Pristiq™ Desvenlafaxine [package insert]. Philadelphia, PA: Wyeth Pharmaceuticals, Inc.; 2009 January.

114. Trazodone [package insert]. Pomona, NY: Barr Laboratories, Inc.; 2008 January.

115. Oleptro™ trazodone [package insert]. Labopharm Europe Limited, Dublin, Ireland, 2010.

116. Nefazodone [package insert]. Sellersville, PA: Teva Pharmaceuticals; 2005 February.

117. Viibryd™, Vilazodone [package insert]. Trovis Pharmaceuticals, LLC. Accessed on 8/22/2012 from http://www.frx.com/pi/viibryd_pi.pdf

118. Remeron® Mirtazapine [package insert]. Organon Inc., West Orange, NJ. 2001.

119. Ables AZ, Nagubilli R. Prevention, recognition, and management of serotonin syndrome. Am Fam Physician.2010 May 1;81(9):1139-42.

120. Dunkley EJ, Isbister GK, Sibbritt D, Dawson AH, Whyte IM (September 2003). "The Hunter Serotonin Toxicity Criteria: simple and accurate diagnostic decision rules for serotonin toxicity". QJM 96 (9): 635–42. doi:10.1093/qjmed/hcg109. PMID 12925718

121. Sternbach H. The serotonin syndrome. Am J Psychiatry. 1991;148:705–713.

122. Ultram® (tramadol) [package insert]. Raritan, NJ; Ortho-McNeil Pharmaceutical, Inc.; 2007 Feb.

123. Keegan MT, Brown DR, Rabinstein AA. Serotonin syndrome from the interaction of cyclobenzaprine with other serotonergic drugs. Anesth Analg 2006;103:1466-8.

124. Silberstein S, Loder E, Diamond S, et al. Probable migraine in the United States: Results of the American Migraine Prevalence and Prevention (AMPP) study. Cephalalgia. 2007;27:220-234.

125. Gillman PK. Triptans, Serotonin Agonists, and Serotonin Syndrome (Serotonin Toxicity): A Review. Headache. 2010 Feb;50(2):264-72. Epub 2009 Nov 17.

126. Leung M, Ong M. Lack of an interaction between sumatriptan and selective serotonin reuptake inhibitors. Headache 1995;35:488-9.

127. Ables AZ and Nagubilli R. Prevention, recognition, and management of serotonin syndrome. *American Family Physician* 2010 May 1;81(9):1139-42.
128. Keegan MT, Brown DR, Rabinstein AA. Serotonin syndrome from the interaction of cyclobenzaprine with other serotoninergic drugs. *Anesth Analg* 2006;103:1466-8.
129. Pigott TA. Gender differences in the epidemiology and treatment of anxiety disorders. *J Clin Psychiatry* 1999;60 Suppl.8:4-15.
130. Professor C Heather Ashton DM, FRCP. Benzodiazepines: How They Work & How to Withdraw. Available at http://benzo.org.uk/manual/bzcha01.htm#26. Accessed on June 23, 2003.
131. Obiora, E, Hubbard R, Sanders RD, *et al.* The impact of benzodiazepines on occurrence of pneumonia and mortality from pneumonia: a nested case-control and survival analysis in a population-based cohort. *Thorax* 2012; doi:10.1136/thoraxjnl-2012-202374.
132. Gold Standard, Inc. Benzodiazepines. Clinical Pharmacology [database online]. Available at: http://www.clinicalpharmacology.com. Accessed: February 2, 2012.
133. Xanax®, alprazolam [package insert]. Pharmacia & Upjohn Company, Kalamazoo, MI, 2003.
134. Librium®, chlordiazepoxide [package insert]. Roche Laboratories, Nutley, NJ, 1995.
135. Tranxene®, clorazepate [package insert]. Ovation Pharmaceuticals. Deerfield, Illinois, 2002.
136. Valium®, diazepam. [package insert]. Roche Pharmaceuticals. Nutley, New Jersey, 2008.
137. Prosom® estazolam [package insert]. Abbott Laboratories, North Chicago, IL, 2006.
138. Paxipam®, halazepam [package insert]. Schering Corp, Kenilworth, NJ, 1990.
139. Ativan®, lorazepam [package insert]. Wyeth pharmaceuticals Inc. Philadelphia, Pennsylvania, 2007.
140. Klonopin® clonazepam [package insert]. Roche Laboratories, Inc., Nutley, NJ, 2001.
141. Serax®, oxazepam [package insert]. Faulding and Wyeth-Ayerst Laboratories, Philadelphia, PA, 2000.
142. Centrax®, prazepam. [package insert]. Parke-Davis, Morris Plains, NJ, 1990.
143. Restoril®, temazepam [package insert]. Mallinckrodt. St. Louis, Missouri, 2007.
144. Halcion®, triazolam. [package insert]. Pharmacia & Upjohn Company. Kalamazoo, Michigan, 2002.
145. Gardner D, Murphy A, O'Donnell H, *et al.* International consensus study of antipsychotic dosing. *Am J Psychiatry*. 2010; 167:686-93.
146. Tauscher J and Kapur S. Choosing the right dose of antipsychotics in schizophrenia: lessons from neuroimaging studies. *CNS Drugs* 2001;15(9):671-8.
147. Agid O, Kapur S, Remington G. Emerging drugs for schizophrenia. *Expert Opinion on Emerging Drugs*. 13(3):479-95, September 2008.
148. Bishara D, Taylor D. Upcoming agents for the treatment of schizophrenia: mechanism of action, efficacy and tolerability. *Drugs*. 68(16):2269-92, May 2008.
149. Farde L, Nyberg S, Oxenstierna G, *et al.* Positron emission tomography studies on D2 and 5-HT2 receptor binding in risperidone-treated schizophrenic patients. *J Clin Psychopharmacol* 1995;15:19SY23S.
150. Kapur S, Zipursky R, Jones C, *et al.* Relationship between dopamine D(2) occupancy, clinical response, and side effects: a double-blind PET study of first-episode schizophrenia. *Am J Psychiatry* 2000;157:514-520.
151. Uchida H, Kapur S, Mulsant BH, *et al.* Sensitivity of older patients to antipsychotic motor side effects: a PET study examining potential mechanisms. *Am J Geriatr Psychiatry* 2009;17:255-263.
152. Uchida H, Kapur S, Pollock BG, *et al.* Optimal dosing of antipsychotic drugs in older patients with schizophrenia: PET investigations. *Int J Neuropsychopharm* 2008;11(suppl 1):136
153. Uchida H, Takeuchi H, Graff-Guerrero A, *et al.* Dopamine D2 receptor occupancy and clinical effects: a systematic review and pooled analysis. *J Clin Psychopharmacology* 2011 Aug;31(4):497-502.
154. Thorazine®, Chlorpromazine [package insert]. Sandoz Inc, Broomfield, CO, 2004.
155. Mellaril®, Thioridazine [package insert]. Novartis Pharmaceuticals Corporation, East Hanover, NJ. 2000.
156. Serentil®, Mesoridazine [package insert]. Novartis Pharmaceuticals Canada Inc, Quebec, Canada, 2000.
157. Moban®, Molindone [package insert]. Endo Pharmaceuticals Inc, Chadds Ford, PA, 2008.
158. Loxitane®, Loxapine [package insert]. Watson Pharma Inc, Corona, CA, 2001.
159. Trilafon®, Perphenazine [package insert]. Schering Corporation, Kenilworth, NJ, 2002.
160. Stelazine®, Trifluoperazine [package insert]. GlaxoSmithKline, Research Triangle Park, NC, 2002.
161. Navane®, Thiothixene [package insert]. Pfizer Inc, NY, NY, 2008.
162. Haldol®, Haloperidol [package insert]. Apotex Inc, Toronto, Canada, 2004.
163. Haloperidol Decanoate [package insert]. Bedford Laboratories™, Bedford, OH 2005.
164. Prolixin®, Fluphenazine [package insert]. Ben Venue Inc, Bedford, OH, 1998.
165. Fluphenazine Decanoate [package insert]. Bedford Laboratories™, Bedford, OH, 2010
166. Clozaril® clozapine [package insert]. Novartis Pharmaceuticals Corporation, East Hanover, NJ, 2008.
167. Fazaclo® clozapine [package insert]. Azur Pharma, Inc, Philadelphia, PA 2010.
168. Devinsky O, Honigfeld G, Patin J. Clozapine-related seizures. *Neurology*. 41:369-371.
169. Perry PJ, Miller DD. The clinical utility of clozapine plasma concentrations. In: Marder SR, Davis JM, Janiack PG(eds). Clinical use of neuroleptic plasma levels. Arlington, VA: American Psychiatric Association. 1993;85-100.
170. Hasegawa M, Guitierrez-Esteinou R, Way L, *et al.* Relationship between clinical efficacy and clozapine concentrations in plasma in schizophrenia: effect of smoking. *J Clin Psychopharmacol*. 1993; 13:83-90.
171. Kronig MH, Munne RA, Szymanski S, *et al.* Plasma clozapine levels and therapeutic response for treatment refractory schizophrenic patients. *Am J Psychiatry*. 1995; 152:179-82.
172. Perry PJ, Miller DD, Arndt SV, *et al.* Clozapine and norclozapine plasma concentrations and clinical response of treatment-refractory schizophrenic patients. *Am J Psychiatry*. 1991; 148:231-5.
173. Potkin SG, Bera R, Gulasekaram B, *et al.* Plasma clozapine concentrations predict clinical response in treatment-resistant schizophrenia. *J Clin Psychiatry*. 1994; 55(Suppl B):133-6.
174. Miller DD, Fleming F, Holman TL, *et al.* Plasma clozapine concentrations as a predictor of clinical response: a follow-up study. *J Clin Psychiatry*. 1994; 55(Suppl B):117-21.
175. Risperdal® risperidone [package insert]. Ortho-McNeil-Janssen Pharmaceuticals Inc, Gurabo, Puerto Rico, 2007.
176. Risperdal® Consta® [package insert]. Janssen Pharmaceuticals, Inc., Titusville, NJ, 2009.
177. Invega® paliperidone [package insert]. ALZA Corporation, Mountain View, CA, 2007.
178. Invega® Sustenna® [package insert]. Janssen Pharmaceuticals, Inc., Titusville, NJ, 2010.

179. Zyprexa® olanzapine [package insert]. Eli Lilly and Company, Indianapolis, IN, 2009.
180. Haslemo T, et al. Valproic Acid Significantly Lowers Serum Concentrations of Olanzapine - An Interaction Effect Comparable With Smoking. Therapeutic Drug Monitoring Oct. 2012;34(5):512-517.
181. Zyprexa® Relprevv™ [package insert]. Eli Lilly and Company, Indianapolis, IN 2009
182. Abilify® aripiprazole [package insert]. Otsuka Pharmaceutical Co. Ltd., Tokyo, Japan, 2008.
183. Saphris® asenapine [package insert]. Merck & Co., Inc., Whitehouse Station, NJ, 2010.
184. Latuda® lurasidone [package insert]. Sunovion Pharmaceuticals, Marlborough, MA 2012.
185. Ihara H, Arai H. Ethical dilemma associated with the off-label use of antipsychotic drugs for the treatment of behavioral and psychological symptoms of dementia. Psychogeriatrics. 8(1):32-37, March 2008.
186. Holt R, Peveler R. Association between antipsychotic drugs and diabetes. Diabetes, Obesity & Metabolism. 8(2):125-135, March 2006.
187. Neil W, Curran S, Wattis J, et al. Antipsychotic prescribing in older people. Age & Aging. 32(5):475-483, September 2003.
188. American Diabetes Association, American Psychiatric Association, American Association of Clinical Endocrinologists, and North American Association for the study of Obesity. Consensus Development Conference on Antipsychotic Drugs and Obesity and Diabetes. Diabetes Care 2004;27(2):596-601).
189. Washington NB, Brahm NC, and Kissack J. Which psychotropics carry the greatest risk of QTc prolongation? Current Psychiatry Oct. 2012;11(10):36-39.
190. David SR, Taylor CC, Kinon BJ, et al. The effects of olanzapine, risperidone, and haloperidol on plasma prolactin levels in patients with schizophrenia. Clinical Therapeutics 2000;22(9):1085-1096.
191. Gray R, Spilling R, Burgess D, et al. Antipsychotic long-acting injections in clinical practice: medication management and patient choice. Br J Psychiatry Suppl. 2009;52:S51-56.
192. Cocoman A, Murray J. Intramuscular injections; a review of best practices for mental health nurses. J Psychiatr Ment Health Nurs. 2008;15(5):424-434.
193. Wynaden D, Landsborough I, McGowans S, et al. Best practice guidelines for the administration of intramuscular injections in the mental health setting. Int J Ment Health Nurs. 2006;15(3):195-200.
194. Eerdekens M, Van Hove I, Remmerie B, et al. Pharmacokinetics and Tolerability of Long-Acting Risperidone in Schizophrenia. Schizophr Res. 2004;70:91-100.
195. Volpicelli JR, Volpicelli LA, O'Brien CP. Medical management of alcohol dependence: clinical use and limitations of naltrexone treatment. Alcohol. 1995 Nov;30(6):789-98.
196. Sees KL. Pharmacological adjuncts for the treatment of withdrawal syndromes. J Psychoactive Drugs. 1991 Oct-Dec;23(4):371-85.
197. Rounsaville BJ. DSM-V research agenda: substance abuse/psychosis comorbidity. Schizophrenia Bulletin. 33(4):947-52, 2007 Jul.
198. Kleber HD. Pharmacologic treatments for opioid dependence: detoxification and maintenance options. Dialogues Clin Neurosci. 2007; 9(4):455-70.
199. Antabuse® disulfiram [package insert]. Barr Pharmaceuticals, L.L.C., Pomona, New York, 2010.
200. Revia® naltrexone [package insert]. Barr Pharmaceuticals, Inc., Pomona, New York, 2009.
201. Vivitrol® naltrexone extended-release injection [package insert]. Alkermes, Inc., Waltham, MA, 2010.
202. Campral® acamprosate [package insert]. Forest Laboratories, Inc., St. Louis, MO, 2004.
203. Suboxone® buprenorphine [package insert]. Reckitt Benckiser Pharmaceuticals, Inc. Richmond, VA.
204. Brahm NC, Yeager LL, Fox MD, et al. Commonly prescribed medications and potential false-positive urine drug screens. Am J Health Syst Pharm 2010 Aug15;67(16):1344-50.
205. Moeller KE, Lee KC, and Kissack JC. Urine Drug Screening: Practical Guide for Clinicians. Mayo Clin Proc.January 2008;83(1):66-76. Available at: www.mayoclinicproceedings.com Accessed on May 23, 2012.
206. Taimapedia. Opioid comparison chart. Last updated September 28, 2011. Available at: http://taimapedia.org/index.php?title=Opioid_comparison_chart. Accessed on May 23, 2012.
207. Cupp M. Equianalgesic dosing of opioids for pain management. Pharmacist's Letter/Prescriber's Letter. August 2012;28(8):280801
208. Antipsychotics drugs class labeling change treatment during pregnancy and potential risk to newborns. Food and Drug Administration, Feb. 2011. http://www.fda.gov/safety/medwatch/safetyinformation/safetyalertsforhumanmedicalproducts/ucm244175.htm.
209. Arnon J, Shechtman S, Ornoy A. The use of psychotropic drugs in pregnancy and lactation. Isr J Psychiatry Relat Sci. 2000;37(3):205-22.
210. Pedersen CA. Postpartum mood and anxiety disorders: a guide for the nonpsychiatric clinician with an aside on thyroid associations with postpartum mood. Thyroid. 1999 Jul;9(7):691-7.
211. Trixler M, Tényi T. Antipsychotic use in pregnancy. What are the best treatment options? Drug Saf. 1997 Jun;16(6):403-10.
212. Kuller JA, Katz VL, McMahon MJ, Wells SR, Bashford RA. Pharmacologic treatment of psychiatric disease in pregnancy and lactation: fetal and neonatal effects. Obstet Gynecol. 1996 May;87(5 Pt 1):789-94.
213. Menon SJ. Psychotropic medication during pregnancy and lactation. Arch Gynecol Obstet 2008 Jan;277(1):1-13.
214. Gentile S. The safety of newer antidepressants in pregnancy and breastfeeding. Drug Saf. 2005;28(2):137-52.
215. Levey L, Ragan K, Hower-Hartley A, et al. Psychiatric disorders in pregnancy. Neurol Clin 2004 Nov;22(4):863-93.
216. Iqbal MM, Aneja A, Fremont WP. Effects of chlordiazepoxide (Librium) during pregnancy and lactation. Conn Med. 2001;39(4):381-92.
217. Iqbal MM, Sobhan T, Aftab SR, Mahmud SZ. Diazepam use during pregnancy: a review of the literature. Del Med J. 2002 Mar;74(3):127-35.
218. El Marroun H. Maternal SSRI Use During Pregnancy: New Findings on Fetal Development. Psychiatry Weekly 2012, May 21, Volume 7, Issue 10 Accessed at http://www.psychweekly.com/aspx/article/articledetail.aspx?articleid=1450 on 6/4/2012.
219. El Marroun, H, Jaddoe VWV, Hudziak JJ, et al. Maternal Use of Selective Serotonin Reuptake Inhibitors, Fetal Growth, and Risk of Adverse Birth Outcomes. Arch Gen Psychiatry. July 2012;69(7):706-714 doi:10.1001/archgenpsychiatry.2011.2333
220. Moretti, M.E., Koren, G., Verjee, Z. & Ito, S. Monitoring lithium in breast milk: An individualized approach for breast-feeding mothers. Therapeutic Drug Monitoring 2003;25(3):364–366.

221. Radley DC, Finkelstein SN, Stafford RS. Off-label prescribing among office based physicians. *Arch Intern Med.* 2006;166:1021-26.
222. Bridge JA, Birmaher B, Iyenger S, *et al.* Placebo response in randomized controlled trials of antidepressants for pediatric major depressive disorder. *American Journal of Psychiatry.* 166(1):42-9, 2009 Jan.
223. Ackermann RT, Williams JW Jr. Rational treatment choices for non-major depressions in primary care: an evidence-based review. *Journal of General Internal Medicine.* 17(4):293-301, 2002 Apr.
224. Tsapakis EM, Soldani F, Tondo L, *et al.* Efficacy of antidepressants in juvenile depression: meta-analysis. *British Journal of Psychiatry.* 193(1):10-7, 2008 Jul.
225. Dubicka B, MRCPsych; Hadley S, Roberts C. Suicidal behavior in youths with depression treated with new-generation antidepressants: Meta-analysis. *British Journal of Psychiatry.* 189(5):393-398, November 2006.
226. Hall WD, Lucke J. How have the selected serotonin reuptake inhibitor antidepressants affected suicide mortality?. *Australian & New Zealand Journal of Psychiatry* 40(11-12): 941-950, November/December 2006.
227. Cheung AH, Emslie GJ, Mayes TL. The use of antidepressants to treat depression in children and adolescents. *CMAJ Canadian Medical Association Journal.* 174(2):193-200, January 17, 2006.
228. Schwenkhagen AM, Stodieck SR. Which contraception for women with epilepsy? *Seizure.* 2008 Mar;17(2):145-50. Epub 2008 Jan 4.
229. Boudreau DM, Yu O, Gray SL, *et al.* Concomitant use of cholinesterase inhibitors and anticholinergics: prevalence and outcomes. *J Am Geriatr Soc.* 2011 Nov;59(11):2069-76. doi: 10.1111/j.1532-5415.2011.03654.x. Epub 2011 Oct 22.
230. Beers MH *et al.* Explicit criteria for determining inappropriate medication use in nursing home residents. *Arch Intern Med* 1991;151:1825-32.
231. The American Geriatrics Society 2012 Beers Criteria Update Expert Panel. American Geriatrics Society Updated Beers Criteria for Potentially Inappropriate Medication Use in Older Adults. *Journal of The American Geriatrics Society* 2012; DOI: 10.1111/j.1532-5415.2012.03923.x. p.1-12.
232. Billioti de Gage S, Begaud B, Bazin F, *et al.* Benzodiazepine use and risk of dementia: prospective population based study. *BMJ* 2012;345:e6231 doi:1136/bmj.e6231 (Published 27 September 2012)
233. Wobrock T, Soyka M. Pharmacotherapy of schizophrenia with comorbid substance use disorder–reviewing the evidence and clinical recommendations. *Progress in Neuro-Psychopharmacology & Biological Psychiatry.* 32(6):1375-85, August 2008.
234. Muller-Vahl K, Emrich H. Cannabis and schizophrenia: towards a cannabinoid hypothesis of schizophrenia. *Expert Review of Neurotherapeutics.* 8(7):1037-48, July 2008.
235. Wells K, Klap R, Koike A, *et al.* Ethnic disparities in unmet need for alcoholism, drug abuse, and mental health care. *Am J Psychiatry.* 2001;158:2027-2032.
236. Gören JL, Parks JJ, and Ghinassi FA, *et al.* When is antipsychotic polypharmacy supported by research evidence? Implications for QI. *The Joint Commission Journal on Quality and Patient Safety* 2008;34(10):571-82.
237. Maglione M, Ruelaz Maher A, Hu J, *et al.* Off-label use of atypical antipsychotics: an update. Comparative Effectiveness Review No. 43. (Prepared by the Southern California/RAND Evidence-based Practice under Contract No. HHSA290-2007-10062-1.) AHRQ Publication No.11-ECH087-EF. Rockville, MD: Agency for Healthcare Research and Quality. September 2011. http://www.effectivehealthcare.ahrq.gov/reports/final.cfm
238. Gugger JJ and Cassagnol M. Low-Dose Quetiapine Is Not a Benign Sedative-Hypnotic Agent. *The American Journal on Addictions* 2008;17:454–455.
239. Correll CU, Rummel-Kluge C, Corves C, *et al.* Antipsychotic Combinations vs Monotherapy in Schizophrenia: A Meta-analysis of Randomized Controlled Trials. *Schizophrenia Bulletin* 2009;35(2):443–457, doi:10.1093/schbul/sbn018.
240. Blier P, Ward HE, Tremblay P, *et al.* Combination of Antidepressant Medications From Treatment Initiation for Major Depressive Disorder: A Double-Blind Randomized Study. *Am J Psychiatry* 2010;167:281-8.
241. Nelson JC, Mazure CM, Jatlow PI, *et al.* Combining norepinephrine and serotonin reuptake inhibition mechanisms for treatment of depression: a double-blind, randomized study. *Biol Psychiatry* 2004;55(3):296-300.
242. Citrome L. Combination Treatments: Your Individual Mileage May Vary. Accessed at www.medscape.com/viewarticle/746887 on 8/9/2011.
243. Julius RJ, Novitsky MA Jr, Dubin WR. Medication adherence: a review of the literature and implications for clinical practice. *J Psychiatr Pract.* 2009;15:34-44.
244. Newcomer JW, Hennekens CH. Severe mental illness and risk of cardiovascular disease. *JAMA.* 2007;298:1794-1796. Abstract
245. Druss BG, Bradford WD, Rosenheck RA, Radford MJ, Krumholz HM. Quality of medical care and excess mortality in older patients with mental disorders. *Arch Gen Psychiatry* 2001;58:565-572.

SUPPLEMENTAL REFERENCES

Adderall® mixed amphetamine salts [package insert]. Wayne, PA: Shire US Inc.; 2011 August.
Ambien® zolpidem [package insert]. Sanofi-Aventis US,LLC, Bridgewater, NJ, 2008.
Amoxapine [package insert]. Corona, CA: Watson Laboratories, Inc.; 2008 June.
Arendt J. Safety in melatonin in long-term use. *J Biol rhythms.* 1997 Dec;12(6):673-81.
Beaudreau S, O'Hara R. Late-Life Anxiety and Cognitive Impairment: A Review. *American Journal of Geriatric Psychiatry.* 16(10):790-803, October 2008.
Benadryl® diphenhydramine [package insert]. Parke-Davis, Morris Plains, NJ, 1999.
Borowsky SJ, Rubenstein LV, Meredith LS, Camp P, Jackson-Triche M, Wells KB. Who is at risk of non-detection of mental health problems in primary care? *J Gen Intern Med.* 2000;15:381-388.
Brown R, Gerbarg P. Herbs and Nutrients in the Treatment of Depression, Anxiety, Insomnia, Migraine, and Obesity. *Journal of Psychiatric Practice.* 7(2):75-91, March 2001.
Clomipramine [package insert]. Hazelwood, MO: Mallinckrodt Inc.; 2007 Mat.
Cook BL, McGuire T, Miranda J. Measuring trends in mental health care disparities, 2000 2004. *Psychiatr Serv.* 2007;58:1533-1540.
Daytrana® methylphenidate patch [package insert]. Shire US Inc., Wayne, PA 2007.
Dextroamphetamine [package insert]. Research Triangle Park, NC: GlaxoSmithKline; 2007 November.

Doxepin [package insert]. New York, NY: Pfizer, Inc.; 2003 October.

Elavil® amitriptyline [package insert]. West Point, PA: Zeneca Pharmaceuticals; 2000 December.

Felbatol® felbamate [package insert]. Wallace Laboratories, Cranbury, NJ, 2000

Freeman EW. Luteal phase administration of agents for the treatment of premenstrual dysphoric disorder. *CNS Drugs.* 2004;18(7):453-68.

Gabitril® tiagabine hydrochloride [package insert]. Cephalon, Inc., West Chester, PA, 2005.

Gerard S. Reviewing medications for bipolar disorder: understanding the mechanisms of action. *Journal of Clinical Psychiatry.* 70(1):e02, 2009 Jan.

Inderal®, propranolol [package insert]. Wyeth Pharmaceuticals, Inc, Philadelphia, PA, 2007.

Leo RJ, Sherry C, Jones AW. Referral patterns and recognition of depression among African-American and Caucasian patients. *Gen Hosp Psychiatry.* 1998;20:175-182.

Lunesta®, eszopiclone [package insert]. Sepracor Inc, Marlborough, MA, 2008.

Maprotiline [package insert].Summit, NJ: Ciba-Geigy Co.; 2006 February.

Melfi C, Croghan T, Hanna M, *et al.* Racial variation in antidepressant treatment in a Medicaid population. *J Clin Psychiatry.* 2000;61:16-21.

Methylphenidate [package insert]. Corona, Ca: Watson Laboratories, Inc.; 2002 July.

Miltown® meprobamate [package insert]. Wallace Laboratories, Cranbury, NJ, 2001

Mysoline® primidone [package insert]. Wyeth-Ayerst Laboratories Inc, Philadelphia, PA, 1995

National Resource Center on ADHD: A program of CHADD, 2008.

Neurontin® gabapentin [package insert]. Pfizer Inc., New York, NY, 2003.

Phenelzine [package insert]. New York, NY: Pfizer, Inc,; 2007 August.

Protriptyline [package insert]. West Point, PA; Merck&Co., Inc.; 1996 July.

Ritalin® methylphenidate [package insert]. Novartis Pharmaceuticals, East Hanover, NJ, 2010.

Schutte-Rodin S, Borch L, Buysse D, *et al.* Clinical guideline for the evaluation and management of chronic insomnia in adults. *J Clin Sleep Med.* 2008; 4(5):487-504.

Sonata® zaleplon [package insert]. Wyeth Laboratories, Philadelphia, PA, 2003.

Tofranil® imipramine [package insert]. Hazelwood, MO: Mallinckrodt Inc.; 2007 September.

Topamax® topiramate [package insert]. Ortho-McNeil Pharmaceutical, Raritan, NJ, 2004.

Tranylcypromine [package insert]. Spring Valley, NY: Par Pharmaceuticals Companies, Inc.; 2007 August.

Trimipramine [package insert].Research Triangle Park, NC: GlaxoSmithKline; 2001 Aug.

Vistaril® hydroxyzine pamoate [package insert]. Pfizer Inc, New York, NY, 2004.

Wilson SJ, Nutt DJ, Alford C, *et al.* British association for psychopharmacology consensus statement on evidence-based treatment of insomnia, parasomnias and circadian rhythm disorders. *J Psychopharmacol.* 2010;24(11):1577-1600.

Zarontin® ethosuximide capsules [package insert]. Parke-Davis Div of Warner-Lambert Co., Morris Plains, NJ, 2000.

INDEX

Alprazolam 5,6,18,19,23,24
Amitriptyline 3,4,8,11
Amoxapine 3,8,17,21,26
Aripiprazole 4,28,29
Armodafanil 8
Asenapine 4,28,29
Atomoxetine 3,13
Benztropine 25
Bupropion 3,13,17,19,21,34,37
Buspirone 4,6,20,23,38
Carbamazepine 2,3,6,7,16,28,34,36,38
Chlordiazepoxide 4,5,6,23,24,31,34
Chlorpromazine 4,26,29,34
Citalopram 3,18
Clomipramine 3
Clonazepam 5,6,23,24
Clonidine 3,10,13,20,23,31
Clorazepate 5,6,23,24
Clozapine 4,26,27,28,29
Desipramine 3,7,8,34,38
Desvenlafaxine 3,8,18,19
Dexmethylphenidate 8,14
Dextroamphetamine 3,8,14
Diazepam 5,6,233,24,25,31,34
Diphenhydramine 4,25,34
Doxepin 3,4,11,36
Duloxetine 3,18,19
Escitalopram 3,8,18
Estazolam 5,24
Eszopiclone 4,8,11
Ethosuximide 3
Fluoxetine 3,4,16,17,18,22,23,37,38
Felbamate 3
Fluphenazine 4,26,29,30
Fluvoxamine 3,18,23
Gabapentin 3,8
Guanfacine 3,13
Halazepam 5
Haloperidol 4,6,25,26,28,29,30
Hydroxyzine 4,24
Iloperidone 4,7,28,29
Imipramine 3,8,34,36
Isocarboxazid 3
Lamotrigine 3,16
Levetiracetam 3
Lisdexamfetamine 3,14
Lithium 3,5,6,7,8,9,15,18,29,36,38
Lorazepam 5,6,23,24,25,31
Loxapine 4,8,26,29
Lurasidone 4,28,29
Maprotiline 3,17,21,36
Meprobamate 4
Mesoridazine 4,8,26,28,29,34
Methylphenidate 3,10,13,14
Mirtazapine 3,6,11,20,21,23,37
Mixed Amphetamine Salts 3,14
Modafinil 3,13
Molindone 4,26,29
Nefazodone 3,11,19,23

Nortriptyline ... 3,7,8,38
Olanzapine ... 3,4,6,16,27,28,29,30,37,38
Oxazepam ... 5,6,23,24,31
Oxcarbazepine ... 3,8,16
Paliperidone ... 4,8,27,28,29,30
Paroxetine ... 3,18,22,23
Perphenazine ... 4,26,29
Phenelzine ... 3,17,21,23
Phenobarbital ... 4,26,29
Phenytoin ... 3,7,16,27,38
Prazepam ... 5,6,23
Prazosin ... 23
Primidone ... 3,16
Propranolol ... 4,18,25
Protriptyline ... 3
Quetiapine ... 4,16,27,28,29,34,37
Ramelteon ... 4,11
Risperidone ... 4,6,8,27,28,29,30
Selegiline ... 3,17,34
Sertraline ... 3,17,18,23,34
Temazepam ... 5,6,23,24,31
Thioridazine ... 4,7,8,26,28,29,34
Thiothixene ... 4,26,29
Tiagabine ... 3
Topiramate ... 3,8
Tranylcypromine ... 3,17,21
Trazodone ... 3,4,11,19,34,38
Triazolam ... 5,18,19,23,24
Trifluoperazine ... 4,26,29
Valproic Acid ... 2,3,5,6,7,9,15,16,27,29,38
Venlafaxine ... 3,8,18,19,34,37
Zaleplon ... 4,11
Ziprasidone ... 4,7,27,28,29
Zolpidem ... 4,11
Zonisamide ... 3

13022742R00030

Made in the USA
San Bernardino, CA
05 July 2014